VALUE-FREEDOM IN SCIENCE AND TECHNOLOGY

HARVARD THEOLOGICAL REVIEW
HARVARD DISSERTATIONS IN RELIGION

edited by

Caroline Bynum

and

George Rupp

Number 8
VALUE-FREEDOM IN SCIENCE AND TECHNOLOGY

by

Robert M. Veatch

SCHOLARS PRESS
Missoula, Montana

VALUE-FREEDOM IN SCIENCE AND TECHNOLOGY:
A Study of the Importance of the Religious, Ethical, and
Other Socio-Cultural Factors in Selected Medical Decisions
Regarding Birth Control

by
Robert M. Veatch

Published by
SCHOLARS PRESS
for
Harvard Theological Review

Distributed by

SCHOLARS PRESS
University of Montana
Missoula, Montana 59801

VALUE-FREEDOM IN SCIENCE AND TECHNOLOGY

by

Robert M. Veatch
Institute of Society, Ethics and Life Sciences
Hastings Center 360 Broadway
Hastings-on-Hudson, New York 10706

Library of Congress Cataloging in Publication Data
Veatch, Robert M
  Value-freedom in science and technology.

  (Harvard dissertations in religion ; no. 8)
  Thesis—Harvard University, 1971.
  Bibliography: p.
  1. Medical ethics. 2. Physician and patient.
3. Birth control—Religious aspects. 4. Decision-
making. 5. Science and ethics. I. Title.
II. Series.
R725.5.V4   176   76-28192
ISBN 0-89130-080-5

Printed in the United States of America
Edwards Brothers, Inc.
Ann Arbor, Michigan 48104

for Paul

PREFACE

Science and values, at once so radically different and so
intimately intertwined, have both staked irrevocable claims on
my life. This volume is an effort to examine this complex
relation. It is a modest reworking of a doctoral dissertation
written in the Religion and Society Program at Harvard University.

The original first chapter has been converted into a brief
introduction to meet editors' requirements. The present first
chapter (which was the second in the original dissertation) has
been revised and shortened somewhat. The remainder of the
volume remains as it originally appeared.

At points in the volume I shall touch upon religious and
philosophical ethics, sociology of values, sociology of medicine, history of science, association theory, and survey research. Only in an inter-disciplinary program such as the one
in Religion and Society would one have the breadth and freedom
to draw upon such disparate fields. To those who have provided
leadership for the program, I am grateful. Most especially to
Professor Ralph B. Potter, who has not only served as advisor
for this dissertation, but was the stimulus for the integration
of sociology and ethics which is reflected in it, I am in heavy
debt. To Professors Arthur J. Dyck and Harvey Cox, with whom
along with Professor Potter I enjoyed a close working relationship as Teaching Fellow at various times while at Harvard, special gratitude is also extended. Their thoughts and advice
have been so thoroughly incorporated into my own throughout
this volume that it has been impossible to give adequate credit. From Professor Dyck I learned that ethical propositions
can neither be fully identified nor fully separated from other
types of scientific statements. From Professor Cox, with whom
I first began to develop the ideas contained in this volume, I
learned to view the scientific and technological process simultaneously sympathetically and critically. Dr. James Luther
Adams, whose spirit is the core of the Religion and Society
Program, also provided inspiration and advice in many stages of

this work. The scientific association discussion in Chapter I
especially bears his imprint, but those who know him will recognize other influences of his teaching throughout.

I have been privileged to have sociology teachers whose
interests have included the religious and ethical aspects of
society. Dr. Stanley King has been of great help in developing
the empirical study of physicians and in stimulating interest
in medical sociology as an exciting field of study. Dr. Renée
C. Fox provided invaluable guidance in developing the integrated theory of a medical action system, as did Dr. Talcott Parsons. The impress of Drs. Robert N. Bellah, David Heer, Donald
Warwick, Herbert Kelman, and Michael Useem will also be found
at various points.

Away from Harvard the medical scientists in my life, especially Drs. Terrine K. Adler, E. Leong Way, and Robert Feather-
stone of the Pharmacology Department of the University of California Medical Center in San Francisco, have given me a scientific perspective which I shall never abandon. At the Institute of Society, Ethics and the Life Sciences I am in the debt
of its Director, Dr. Daniel Callahan, not only for making time
available so freely to finish this work, but for the continual
discussion of the subject matter and intellectual stimulation
in an environment which is a living demonstration of the in-
separability of the scientific and the ethical. Also at the
Institute, Sharmon Sollitto and Thomas F. Draper played important roles, as have Leslie English and Patricia Pierce.

Appreciation for the typing of various drafts of this work
is gratefully given to Mrs. Betty Gaylin, Mrs. Edna Moritz,
Mrs. Ada Ishii and Mrs. Marilyn Shemenowski. Finally, to my
wife, Laurelyn Veatch, who has been my intellectual and emotional companion, who has shared in the writing of the theory
and the programing of the computers, but for whom life itself
is ethics, appreciation will never be adequately expressed.

To all of these, if they do not accept the uses I have
made of their ideas I am, of course, alone responsible. If I
forever appear schizophrenic, simultaneously scientist and
philosopher-ethicist, it is because I remain convinced that the
two roles are truly inseparable.

TABLE OF CONTENTS

INTRODUCTION

SCIENCE AND VALUES: AN AMBIGUOUS RELATION

We are currently in the midst of the latest skirmish in history's ongoing struggle over the place of values in science and technology. It is as if there were two battle strategies rooted in two basically different views of reality. Student radicals and their elder brethren are accusing the scientific establishment of hiding behind the shield of "value-freedom" in defense of "pure science," avoiding the social problems of the day. The defenders of "pure science," on the other hand, charge that social activists, by insisting that science must be the servant of values, are, in fact, traitors in the battle, sabotaging the one weapon powerful enough to conquer the problems which are the real enemy of humanity.

While the issues at stake are by no means new, it is no accident that the dispute over the place of values in science and technology, the *Werturteilsstreit*, as the Germans call it, has become critical and explicit during the twentieth century, the period when science has emerged as a colossal automaton with enormous and clearly demonstrated power to affect the conditions of society. The emergence of the technological era casts the *Werturteilsstreit* in a new light. Not only is it now believed that science is capable of solving any problem society is able to pose, but the troops in the service of the colossus are much further removed from the masses of society. There is thus little common understanding of or control over the operations of the technological system. This factor is central in the renewed sense of urgency that attends the subject.

There are two closely related questions in the dispute over the relationship of science and values. First, are values to be included in the category of natural phenomena which can be investigated scientifically, or are they completely outside the realm of the scientific enterprise (except perhaps as phenomenological objects for sociological study)? In short, one question is whether the "ought" can be derived from the "is."

1

Second, is it possible, ideally if not in practice, to exclude values from scientific and technological activity? These two issues, both part of the fact-value controversy, are more closely interconnected than first appears. They both depend on the ontological and epistemological status of values and their relation to (other kinds of) facts.

The dispute can be considered a peculiarly modern phenomenon which had its origin in the late nineteenth and early twentieth centuries when scientists such as Max Weber and Werner Sombart defended the concept of *Werturfreiheit* against the insistence that scientists should be pressed into the service of the state. It can be also seen, in a larger context, as having a much earlier origin. The problem then appears as the relationship between two broad categories: the scientific, the descriptive, the material, the natural, the instrumental, the profane on the one hand and the religious, the prescriptive, the transcendent, the supernatural, the non-material, the non-instrumental, the sacred on the other.

The history of the relationship of science to religion has been seen in evolutionary terms as the gradual emergence of science to replace irrational, superstitious and primitive religious thinking.[1] This view is probably too simple. At least some readings of the so-called primitive societies suggest that simple scientific interpretations of daily tasks such as the provision of shelter and food are already developed and exist alongside of magical and religious belief systems.[2] Just when science is seemingly secure from the encroachment of magic, other-worldly spirituality, the authority of a decadent tradition, or the demands of a particular political system, movements arise which challenge its autonomy. While philosophical dualisms attempt to separate science from the non-scientific, monistic interpretations of reality call the dualisms into check whenever the separation obscures the interpenetration and interrelation of the two spheres. We of the technological era are sufficiently *homo scientificus* that we tend to value the dualistic approach. We view history through scientific spectacles, praising Hippocrates for his differentiation of rational techniques in the observation of illness and cure

from the magico-religious elements of early Greek medical practice. We stand with Galileo on trial for crimes against the
Church and wince when he recants, surrendering his scientific
observations to the authority of the Pope. It may be, however, that the dualists' point has been made, and we need once
again to focus on the points of contact between the scientific
and the evaluative and expressive.

Separating the Scientific and the Evaluative

Throughout history there has been a dialectic between
those who want to separate science from the religious, ethical,
and aesthetic and those who refuse to permit this compartmental
dualism. My objective in this introduction is to sketch the
various forms this separating and combining may take, to construct and exemplify a typology which will be developed in
later chapters of this volume. Without attempting to provide a
detailed historical survey we can identify examples of the attempt to separate the scientific and the religious, evaluative,
and ethical throughout Western thought. For example, in sixth
and fifth century Greek culture the Ionians tended to reject
the explanation of the universe in terms of the mystical and
religious. They attempted to explain the constituents of the
universe not by belief in anthropomorphic gods, but through a
search for its ultimate constituents conceived in terms of material substance, force, and movement. Their method focused on
careful observation, data collection, and cautious generalization. Anaximander's theory of a primal, corporeal substance
was a radical materialistic dualism.[3] Natural substances were
separated from the whims and passions of the human-like gods
with unpredictable inclinations. Knowledge obtained by scientific methods, albeit rudimentary, came to be viewed as an end
in itself.

This pattern of the separation of the scientific and the
evaluative provides the background for the value-free science
controversy of the twentieth century. The development of the
rationalist, relativist, and secularist spirit with the
Enlightenment is its immediate precursor. The modern Western,
especially American, conception of values is derived from the

British empirical philosophy of Locke, which has its roots in the physics or so-called natural science theories of Descartes, Galileo, and Newton. Descartes divided reality into *res extensa* and *res cogitans*, the two heterogeneous categories of body and mind with their own intrinsic natures. In contrast with Augustine, Thomas, and Luther, the polarization is now within the secular world. This fundamental shift opens the way for values to be reduced to secondary interest. The non-material, vectorial element had been preserved until this point as a divinely originating spiritual force. Now the non-material is loosed in an independent, secular sphere, and it fares poorly at the hands of the scientifically oriented modern.

While he rejected Descartes's rationalism, Locke, drawing on Descartes along with the physics of Galileo and Newton, developed the basic duality of extended and thinking substances into empirical philosophy by the separation of primary and secondary. Primary qualities are "utterly inseparable from the body," including measurable, quantifiable phenomena: "solidity, extension, figure, motion or rest, and number." Secondary qualities "in truth are nothing in the objects themselves," including colors, sounds, tastes, etc.[4] Matter has extension and quantifiability, which provide certain perceptions with an objective basis. Other perceptions, while they are projected onto the real world, have no objective existence. This separation reduced the scientific enterprise to those areas which were subject to quantification and mathematical manipulation.

It is a simple step for values and ethical judgments to be relegated to the realm of the subjective in the sense of being mere projections onto physical objects.

There are at least three ways one might separate the scientific and the unscientific. First, the attitude of disinterested atheism or agnosticism with regard to religion, exemplified by the Sophist, Protagoras. In his book *On the Gods* Protagoras remarks:

> With regard to the gods, I cannot know whether
> they exist or do not exist, nor what they are
> like in form; for the factors preventing scien-
> tific knowledge are many: the obscurity of the
> subject, and the shortness of life.[5]

Second, the view that science and religion are thoroughly distinct, and what is significant in life is independent of the scientific enterprise. This attitude is sometimes seen in the neo-Pythagoreans and in post-Galenic medicine which was dominated by the prevailing spirit of magic and mysticism. Ambrose's attitude was that "to discuss the nature and position of the earth does not help us in our hope of the life to come."[6] The position has existed throughout history down to the anti-scientific fundamentalism of the contemporary period.

A third form, a true dualistic separation, could be characterized by the attitude that while the scientific and the nonscientific are utterly distinct, both are meaningful and important. Much of the Hippocratic corpus, particularly *The Sacred Disease*, exemplifies this view. *The Sacred Disease* dating from the fifth century,[7] attacks the notion that epilepsy, or perhaps some other forms of seizures and insanity,[8] is to be distinguished from other diseases by its sacred origin. The author's view about the so-called sacred disease is clear:

> It is not, in my opinion, any more divine or more
> sacred than other diseases, but has a natural
> cause, and its supposed divine origin is due to
> men's inexperience, and to their wonder at its
> peculiar character.[9]

This does not mean, however, that for the Greek physician, the spiritual and divine are not significant. In contrast to the rather small group of agnostic and atheistic philosophers, most held a much more complex position, affirming the gods, but compartmentalizing their theology so that it does not directly affect the scientific aspects of their work.[10] For the Hippocratic physician nature is divine, but this does not imply that the gods intervene directly in the processes of natural illness and healing which are the responsibility of the physician. According to Edelstein, "The two spheres of the divine and of the natural are...fundamentally separate, although their influence is combined in every action."[11] In several of the Hippocratic works including the *Prognostic* and *Decorum* there are suggestions that the divine is reflected in those elements of disease which have traditionally been attributed to magic, spirits, or

other supernatural powers.[12] According to at least some portions of the Corpus dreams are divine and have relevance to
diseases which have an element of the divine, but there is a
complete role separation. The interpretation of the dreams is
properly left to "those who possess the art of dealing with
such things," i.e., the priests.[13] The fourth book on *Regimen*
is devoted to the discussion of dreams, prayers and incanta-
tions and makes clear the division of labor between the religious specialist and the physician. Prayer, according to the
author, "indeed is good, but while calling on the gods a man
should himself lend a hand."[14] Religious medicine is, thus,
not rejected by the Hippocratic physician, although he sees it
as something entirely separate from his realm of competence.

Integrating the Scientific and the Evaluative

While history is full of attempts to isolate the scientific from the religious, emotive, and evaluative, there has always been an opposing force, one which attempts to collapse the
dualism. These integrative stances might be divided into two
types, which I will call "professional" and "radical."

One of the characteristics of a profession is that knowledge and skill in a specific technical area are combined with a
set of norms internal to the profession, which establish a
standard for appropriate behavior in the professional role.
The profession is usually given the responsibility for developing and enforcing these norms. The Hippocratic Oath is a clas-
sic example of this integration of technical skill and normative framework. The Oath, together with two or three other
works of the Corpus, are as different from the treatises we
have been discussing as the modern biochemistry text is from
the American Medical Association's Code of Ethics. They origi-
nate from entirely different philosophical schools. It is the
Oath which provides a good example of the professional integrationist position.

While the earlier works of the Corpus have much in common
with the Ionian perspective, the Oath has been identified by
Edelstein, in the definitive essay on its philosophical origins, as standing explicitly in the Pythagorean tradition.[15]

For the Pythagoreans the scientific was inseparably bound up with the cathetic, evaluative, metaphysical, and religious. As a community they were committed to the search for truth, the quest for religious salvation, and the zeal for moral reformation of the society. There was no radical separation of the material from the sensory, matter from Spirit, fact from feeling or value. Religion and science were two components of an integrated world view. The Oath contains two well differentiated components, a covenant and an ethical code. The covenant[16] is sworn in the name of Apollo, Asclepius, Health (Hygieia), Panacea, and "all the gods and goddesses." In it the young Hippocratic physician swears to hold his teacher as his own parent, to share his income with him, to teach his teacher's children without fee, and to refuse to reveal his knowledge to those outside the familial guild or society. He will guard his life and art in "purity and holiness." This is uniquely characteristic of the Pythagorean brotherhood of the fourth century,[17] going far beyond the level of merely mastering technical knowledge and skills; it introduces a major ethical dimension. The physician will apply his dietetic measures for the benefit of the sick, keeping them from "harm and injustice."[18] He will not participate in euthanasia, abortions or surgery. None of these ethical rules can be reduced to "purely scientific" interests, but rather each is grounded in the Pythagorean philosophical-ethical perspective, which requires not only the ethical life, but also that the scientific enterprise be combined with and incorporated into the larger quest for salvation.

This notion of a peculiar set of ethical norms for an elite professional group of "holy" men is entirely consistent with entrance into this restricted brotherhood through an oath pledging never to divulge its "holy secrets." For the physician who adhered to the Hippocratic Oath, medicine was a unique profession practiced by the members of a unique quasi-religious brotherhood.

The differentiation of a unique set of norms and a unique set of ethical sensitivities which we have called a "professional" ethic is also exemplified in the treatise *On Remedies* by the physician, Scribonius Largus, in the first century A.D.

He identifies the characteristics sympathy (*misericordiae*) and
humanness (*humanitatis*) seemingly to the exclusion of other
ethical norms as the peculiar ethical responsibility of the
medical role. The true physician "is not allowed to harm any-
body, not even the enemies of the state. He may fight against
them with every means as a soldier or as a good citizen,"[19] but
in his role as a physician he must not harm them. Such an ap-
proach--that of professional integration--represents one clas-
sic way of relating ethics and values to the scientific enterprise, in an integrative rather than separationist mode.

The other class of integrative thinking, which I have
termed "radical," goes further, not limiting the synthesis of
science and values to a professional framework. At its best,
it culminates in the view that man is an integrated personality
irrevocably bound to a human community, which brooks no separation of roles or ontological categories such as body and soul.
At its worst, it means the collapse of any distinction between
scientific and the magical and a reversion to the earlier view
of reality in which all events of nature are considered supernatural acts of the spirits. On the level of ethics, a radical
integration requires the rejection of any professional set of
norms in favor of the development of a universalistic normative
ethic applicable to decision-making processes even within the
scientific context.

As an example of a more radical form of integration we
might cite Plato although admittedly his ethical theory is ambiguous. It contains some elements of a more radical form of
integration. It seems clear that he links the virtues to all
social activity including the scientific. Possibly his differentiation of virtues would lead to the development of a "professional ethic" but there is also evidence that the virtues
are not particularized in relation to particular professions.[20]

His theory of the soul and the relationship of virtues to
it provides the strongest evidence that Plato held the position
of radically integrating universalized virtues into a human
ethic, a universal theory of the good.

The virtues of the individual are analogous to those of the state. To initiate his discussion of the virtues of the individual, Plato asks the rhetorical question:

> And so of the individual; we may assume that he has the same three principles in his own soul which are found in the State; and he may be rightly described in the same terms, because he is affected in the same manner?[21]

These patterns of separating and integrating have been repeated in history responding to pressures and excesses of the day. By the beginning of the twentieth century value freedom in science and technology had emerged as a norm required of anyone engaged in the scientific enterprise. The dichotomizing, however, can go only so far before it reaches the limits of internal inconsistency and philosophical implausibility. The integrating forces have emerged once again to demand a much closer relation between science and values. In this volume we shall explore this value-free science controversy, looking first at the debate in the twentieth century science associations, and then attempting a more analytical construction of the relation of values to the scientific enterprise, arguing that it is logically necessary for values to be considered not only in the selection of topics and the application of science to social problem-solving, but in the scientific stage itself.

Part II is a case study of the relation of values to the scientific enterprise. We examine physicians' values regarding oral contraception and, in a sample survey, document how these impinge on scientific judgments and clinical practice. The value interactions between a smaller group of physicians and their patients are explored. We conclude that value freedom is both practically and logically impossible in the scientific enterprise. For scientists, lay people, and society as a whole to fail to realize this and thus fail to establish proper safeguards is both irrational and dangerous.

NOTES

INTRODUCTION

[1]Auguste Comte, *Cours de philosophie positive*, 4th ed.
(6 vols.; Paris, Bailliere, 1877). See also an abridged
translation published as *The Positive Philosophy of Auguste
Comte*, trans. by Harriet Martineau (3 vols.; London: Bell,
1896).

[2]Bronislaw Malinowski, *Magic, Science, and Religion and
Other Essays* (Garden City, New York: Doubleday and Company,
Inc., 1948), pp. 17-92.

[3]See Kathleen Freeman, *Pre-Socratic Philosophers* (Cambridge: Harvard University Press, 1946), pp. 56-58.

[4]*Locke Selections*, ed. by Sterling P. Lamprecht, (New
York: Charles Scribner's Sons, 1928), pp. 205-06.

[5]Protagoras, *On the Gods*, cited in Freeman, *Pre-Socratic
Philosophers*, p. 347.

[6]St. Ambrose cited in F.N.L. Poynter and K. D. Keele, *A
Short History of Medicine* (London: Mills and Boon, 1961), p.
23.

[7]Hippocrates, Jones, ed., *The Sacred Disease*, II, 134.

[8]See *Ibid.*, p. 132.

[9]*Ibid.*, p. 139.

[10]*Ibid.*, p. 208.

[11]Edelstein, "Greek Medicine--Religion and Magic," p. 216.

[12]See Hippocrates, II, Jones, ed., *Decorum*, 289. Cf.
Edelstein, "Greek Medicine--Religion and Magic," pp. 216-17.

[13]Hippocrates, IV, Jones, ed., *Regimen*, IV, 423.

[14]*Ibid.*

[15]Edelstein, "The Hippocratic Oath: Text, Translation, and
Interpretation," in *Ancient Medicine*, pp. 3-63.

[16]Hippocrates, I, Jones, ed., *The Oath*, 299, lines 1-14.

[17]Edelstein, "The Hippocratic Oath," p. 43.

[18]Hippocrates, I, Jones, ed., *The Oath*, 299, lines 16-17.
Jones' translation uses the terms "dietetic measures, injury or
wrong doing." We have followed Edelstein's translation "harm
or injustice." The first three categories of medicine

11

specifically dealt with in the text, dietary measures, drugs, and surgery, are, according to Aristoxenus, those of Pythagorean medicine and in Pythagorean medicine they were dealt with in that order. See Edelstein, "The Hippocratic Oath," p. 21. Jones' translation which generalizes dietetic measures to "treatments" loses this parallel.

Note that the code does not make the prevention of harm by itself the physician's moral duty, as many a modern physician will maintain. It is not a purely utilitarian ethic but a mixed deontological position. The physician is to prevent harm *and injustice*.

[19] Scribonius Largus, *On Remedies*, p. 2, cited in Edelstein's "Ethics of the Greek Physician," p. 338.

[20] In spite of the fact that Plato's theory of the State does not permit association of the virtues of Temperance and Justice to particular class groups, it could still be argued that they form the basis of a class-oriented particularism with regard to ethical responsibility; they both support differentiation of a social division of labor which is ontologically grounded. Temperance is "the agreement of the naturally superior and inferior as to the right rule of either..." Likewise, the Platonic concept of Justice supports differentiation of ethical responsibility: Justice is "everyone doing his own work."

[21] *Ibid.*, IV, 435C, p. 163.

PART I

A THEORETICAL FORMULATION OF THE PLACE

OF VALUES IN SCIENCE AND TECHNOLOGY

CHAPTER I

SCIENCE AND VALUES IN CONTEMPORARY SCIENCE ASSOCIATIONS

In the Introduction we outlined the battle between those
whose task in history focused on drawing lines ever more sharp-
ly between the scientific, the descriptive, the material, and
the religious, the prescriptive, the non-material and those
whose mission was drawing these spheres more closely together.
We suggested that these countervailing tendencies of dichotomizing and integrating were analogous in the history of thought
to the contemporary dispute over the relation of values to the
scientific and technological enterprises. We shall limit ourselves in this chapter to a more detailed account of the *Werturteilsstreit* as it has been reflected in the scientific associations which have emerged with modern science. We shall look
particularly at the associations of the nineteenth and twentieth centuries, concentrating on American associations.

The listing of professional scientific, technical, and
health societies in the United States alone covers over one
hundred fifty pages in the Encyclopedia of Associations. Re-
viewing each would be impossible in our limited space. We have
had to limit our attention to major associations. To provide
some focus for the account we shall pay special attention to
the sociological associations. Due to the nature of their
work, they have often had the value-question come to the surface and dealt explicitly with the arguments. We shall, however, include examples from other associations where applicable. Our analysis leads to the conclusion that there are
three main views on the place of values in science and technology which characterize different groups. The first type we
shall call the pure science association. Like the scientific
works of the Hippocratic corpus they draw sharp divisions between the scientific and the non-scientific. In contrast, the
second type, the applied science associations, have a definite
integrating thrust. Like the Pythagoreans who swore to the
Hippocratic Oath, these groups maintain their unique professional perspective in the integrative efforts. Finally there
are those groups which demand a radical integration.

15

Values mean very different things to these different types of groups. None of them excludes values from the scientific and technological enterprises totally, though the pure scientists often give that impression. None of them totally reduces science and technology to nothing more than values, although the radicals upon occasion come dangerously close. In Chapter IV we shall discuss the many ways in which values are related to science and technology.

The types of solutions to the value-dispute as expressed by varying professional groupings within each discipline appear, among other things, to be chronology dependent. The early American scientific associations, and modern associations more generally, are difficult to classify. They tended to integrate natural scientific pursuits with the broader quest for knowledge, culture, and the good. No sharp distinctions were drawn between scientific and artistic, ethical, or policy concerns. No clear conception of the scientific professional existed. Many of the great contributors to science both in the United States and Europe were clergymen, politicians, and social leaders.

Increase Mather was the leader of the Boston Philosophical Society, the first learned and scientific society organized in the American colonies. Cotton Mather, his son, was a member of the Royal Society of London as were John Winthrop, Roger Williams, Benjamin Franklin, and other cultural figures from the colonies. Jonathan Edwards was the author of the first and only published paper of the Connecticut Society of Arts and Sciences, a treatise "On the Language of the Muhhekaneen Indians."

Scientific societies can be traced back to Plato's academy. They emerged in the modern world, however, in the sixteenth century in Renaissance Italy. In the seventeenth century they were organized throughout Europe and began to develop in the colonies of the new world.[1]

In 1727 Benjamin Franklin organized a literary and scientific society called the Junto. Like the religio-scientific guild of Hippocratic physicians, the Junto was a secret society. It was devoted to mutual improvement in the areas of

morals, politics, and natural philosophy.[2] Although the separation of moral and natural philosophy was maintained, no
sharp lines were drawn.

In 1743 Franklin suggested the formation of the American
Philosophical Society in a letter entitled "A Proposal for Promoting Useful Knowledge among the British Plantations in America." Like its predecessor, there was a thorough mixture of
the natural and moral sciences. They discussed questions of
"natural philosophy, moral science, history, politics," and
carried on investigations in "botany, medicine, mineralogy,
mining, mathematics, chemistry, the arts, trades, and manufac-
tures."[3]

The second half of the eighteenth century was to see
countless societies of this type emerge on American soil, many
of them local in nature. They all were characterized by the
lack of any sharp divisions in their purposes and subject matter, having practical problem-solving in mind. They pursued
the questions of moral philosophy and the finer arts of cultured gentlemen. One of the more important of these groups included the American Society for Promoting and Propagating Useful Knowledge which resulted from the reorganization of the
Junto in 1766.

This period of highly integrated societies of cultured
generalists lasted throughout the first half of the nineteenth
century. There were no permanent national scientific societies
during this period. American scientists, such as they were,
were for the most part either amateur or devoted to practical
problem solving in the service of the government.[4]

The second half of the century saw the emergence of the
more specialized sciences and the development of the attitude
of professionalism. The movement toward pure science associations began by the gathering of scientific disciplines in increasingly specialized groups. Thirteen insane asylum super-
intendents formed the American Psychiatric Association in 1844.
The American Medical Association organized in 1847, the American Association for the Advancement of Science in 1848, but the
development of pure science as a cause which had to be separated, isolated, and defended against the encroachment of values

took time to build reaching its climax in the two decades at
the turn of the century.

THE PURE SCIENCE ASSOCIATIONS

It is the purpose (of the Society) to advance
sociological knowledge by undertaking purely
scientific investigations and surveys, and by
publishing and supporting purely scientific
studies....It rejects all concern with practical
(ethical, religious, political, esthetic, etc.)
goals of any kind.[5]

Deutsche Gesellschaft für Soziologie Statutes

Hippocratic medicine has been described not as opposing
religion and ethics, but as radically separating the scientific
and the religious. This theory of the double truth was secularized in the modern period by the separation of the study of
"objective" physical reality from the merely subjective. This
dualism characterizes the pure scientific associations we have
investigated. The positivist philosophical tradition, at least
in its extreme forms, argues for the utter separation of fact
and value. Weber expresses this dualism when, in his paper on
"The Meaning of 'Ethical Neutrality' in Sociology and Economics," which grew out of the *Werturteilsstreit* of the Verein für
Sozialpolitik, he makes clear that:

What is really at issue is the intrinsically simple
demand that the investigator and teacher should
keep unconditionally separate the establishment of
empirical facts (including the "value-oriented"
conduct of the empirical individual whom he is
investigating) and *his* own practical evaluations,
i.e., his evaluation of these facts as satisfactory
or unsatisfactory (including among these facts
evaluations made by the empirical persons who are
the objects of investigation).[6]

We have selected two primary examples of "pure science"
associations: the Deutsche Gesellschaft für Soziologie as characterized by Max Weber's writings and the American Sociological
Association exemplified by the *American Sociological Review*
editorial policy as stated in 1939.

Weber joined the Verein für Sozialpolitik in the early
1890's giving his maiden speech before the association at its
Berlin meetings in 1893.[7] In the course of the next quarter

century he was to become the major spokesman for a carefully reasoned separation of social science and social policy.[8] The *Verein für Sozialpolitik* was founded in 1872 when Weber was eight years old under the leadership of the great German social economists Gustav Schmoller and Adolf Wagner. This early association did not draw hard lines between objective science and social policy. The *Verein*'s founding charter had included such goals as:

> "supporting the prosperous development" of industry "stimulating timely, well-considered state intervention to protect the just interests of all participants" in the economy, and helping to accomplish "the supreme tasks of our time and our nation."[9]

The *Verein*, in its early years, was dominated by scholar-politicians who helped formulate and who supported Bismarck's welfare state policies.[10] Weber's ambition was to separate scientific pursuit from the policy interests of the Bismarckian Reich. It was in this context that in 1904 Weber, along with Edgar Jaffee and Werner Sombart, took over the editorship of the *Archiv für Sozialwissenschaft und Sozialpolitik*. Their initial statement entitled "'Objectivity' in Social Science and Social Policy" came from Weber's pen. A statement of editorial policy for the *Archiv*, it is one of the classical expositions of what has become known as the "value-free sociology." In many ways it is a more sophisticated precursor to Bain's editorial position paper for the *American Sociological Review*. The Weberian position is that man as scientist should limit his concerns to ideally value-free treatment of "facts" while as citizen he should be responsibly concerned with social policy. Weber announces his editorial policy will be that:

> In the pages of this journal, especially in the discussion of legislation, there will inevitably be found social *policy*, i.e., the statement of ideals, in addition to social *science*, i.e., the analysis of facts. But we do not by any means intend to present such discussions as "science" and we will guard as best we can against allowing these two to be confused with each other....In other words, it should be made explicit just where the arguments are addressed to the analytical understanding and where to the sentiments.[11]

This became the first round in the great *Werturteilsstreit* which was to give rise to the founding of the Deutsche Gesellschaft für Soziologie in 1909. The 1910 statutes of the Gesellschaft state unequivocally:

> It is the purpose (of the Gesellschaft) to advance sociological knowledge by undertaking purely scientific investigations and surveys and by publishing and supporting purely scientific studies....It rejects all concern with practical (ethical, religious, political, esthetic, etc.) goals of any kind.[12]

The dispute reached a climax with an intense debate in January of 1914 between the "pure" and "practical" scientists. Weber's paper for this debate was eventually published as "The Meaning of 'Ethical Neutrality' for Sociology and Economics." The Deutsche Gesellschaft für Soziologie claimed that:

> In contrast to the Verein für Sozialpolitik, whose very purpose is to make propaganda for certain ideals, our purpose has nothing to do with propaganda, but is exclusively one of objective research.[13]

The pure science associations in the social sciences date roughly from the period of this value dispute. The Institut International de Sociologie was founded in Paris in 1894, the Sociological Society of London dates from 1905. The American Sociological Society (now the Association) from 1905.[14] The American Psychological Association was founded in 1892.[15]

The natural science and engineering associations had been evolving over the last half of the nineteenth century. Along with the Psychiatric and Medical Associations and the American Association for the Advancement of Science in the 1840's were the American Society of Civil Engineers (1852), The American Institute of Architects (1857), American Chemical Society (1876), American Society of Mechanical Engineers (1880), Institute of Electrical and Electronic Engineers (1884), American Physiological Society (1887), American Society for Microbiology (1899), American Society of Biological Chemists (1906), American Society for Pharmacology and Experimental Therapeutics (1908), American Institute of Chemical Engineers (1909), American Psychoanalytic Association (1911), American Society for

Experimental Pathology (1913), and the American Association of
Immunologists (1914).

Viewed sociologically, the key to understanding the pure
science associations is their belief in the ability to maintain
a strict separation of roles between scientist and citizen.
Separation is related to their handling of the value-dispute.
In "Science as a Vocation" Weber insists on value-freedom in
the classroom while at the same time recognizing the right and
even the duty of the same individual, as a citizen, to participate in practical politics.[16]

The 1939 editorial position of the *American Sociological
Review* reflects the same standpoint:

> Normative values relating to research methods and
> results are the only ones which the scientist *qua*
> scientist can promote....The scientist as citizen
> in a democracy should play a responsible part in
> this political process, but he should make it
> clear that he is a citizen, not a *scientist*, when
> he does.[17]

A sociological correlate of this strict role separation is
the rigid limitation of membership to holders of doctorates in
the field or a closely related one while students in the field
are permitted student or associate memberships.

The views of the "pure scientists" on the value-dispute
are closely related to this role separation. The "pure scientists," at least if they are pushed at all, do not deny the
necessary presence and importance of the pre-scientific factors. The pure scientists recognize that, for the scientist,
the scientific enterprise is considered valuable and that
values are a necessary part of selecting the topics for scientific study. Weber's term for this phenomenon is value-relevance (*Wertbeziehung*). The problems of the empirical disciplines, he says, are to be solved non-evaluatively, but "the
problems of the social sciences are selected by the value relevance of the phenomena treated."[18] For Weber science was a
"calling." He called it a "terminological misunderstanding"
that his opponents in the *Verein* thought he was saying either
that scientific results were not valuable or that selection of
subject matter did not require evaluation.[19] What *is* unique at
this level is that the pure scientists place relatively strong

emphasis upon the basic value of Truth or Knowledge. According to Marianne Weber's biography, Weber considered freedom of the intellect to be the highest good.[20]

Even in what is more narrowly thought of as a scientific activity, Weber never denied that values are the legitimate subject matter for scientific study. He states his frustration that an

> almost inconceivable misunderstanding which con-
> stantly recurs is that the propositions which I
> propose imply that empirical science cannot treat
> "subjective" evaluations as the subject matter
> of its analysis....[21]

The heart of the pure scientist's fight for value-freedom as the essential ideal of science is their effort to eliminate bias and distortion. Lester F. Ward, in the first presidential address to the American Sociological Society in 1906, illustrates that in their early days the pure social science organizations were deeply involved in trying to demonstrate that the social sciences were indeed sciences,[22] and the heart of modern science is the attempt to eliminate personal or social bias and distortion from the execution of methods and the recording and reporting of data.

During this period the medical sciences were undergoing a similar crisis. The Flexner Report, issued in 1910, made a strong case that medicine had to be placed on a scientific foundation. Medicine until this time was a hodge-podge of folk remedy, unverified tradition, and occasionally bio-medical science. The Flexner Report epitomized for the medical sciences the same drive we have traced for the social sciences: a vigorous crusade to establish a "purely scientific" force free of superstitions, biases, distortions, and the hopes and needs of clients, as the rational foundation of problem solving. It is really at this point that the pure scientists make their case for value-freedom, and most of us are still willing to grant them the crucial significance of the point in the light of the contemporary critiques of value-freedom.

To our knowledge no pure scientist ever claimed that value-freedom was in fact obtained, at least in the sense of eliminating bias and distortion. They held and continue to

hold it as an ideal. They are often guilty, however, of minimizing the attention given to this deviation from the norm.
Parsons and Weber, among others, devote so much attention to
describing the ideal that little effort is made in discussing
procedures for coping with the real, less than ideal world. We
call this tendency to behave as if the ideal were established
(even though one gives verbal recognition to its absence) the
"first fallacy of the ideal-type." This will be elaborated in
Chapter IV.[23]

It is important to realize that this is the context of the
classical statements of the need to separate so-called scientific facts from "mere" values and preferences. The immediate
challenge to Weber and to Flexner was the contamination of descriptive observation and recording by hoped-for outcomes:
whether they be politically expedient policies or hoped-for
cures for incurable diseases. As in the scientific writings of
the Hippocratic treatises the mission of the hour was to make
distinctions where distinctions had to be made.

In this context it is not altogether fair to accuse the
early Hippocratic writers or Weber or Flexner of denying the
existence of points of contact between science and evaluation.
It is true that these men spend little if any time acknowledging that even within the scientific stage values may play a
part. Even within the scientific activity choices must be made
and made routinely; these require a value framework. Even
within the scientific stage procedure is subject to moral evaluation. They may be morally praiseworthy, neutral, or objec-
tionable. If the pure scientists have a blind spot here it is
because they are facing another direction fighting a battle on
a different flank. They are so zealous in excluding bias and
distortion that these other factors are given very little attention.

As we come to the application stage we reach the real crux
of the pure scientist's case for value-freedom. We have already seen that he holds the prerequisites for the radical separation of the scientific and application stages. He believes
in the possibility of a role separation between the scientist
and the citizen; he affirms the priority or at least high

position of the value of Truth; he stresses the value inputs
from bias and distortion which ideally should be eliminated
while he minimizes those which cannot be, i.e., method and
other choices and moral evaluation of the scientific enterprise.

There are at least three possible reasons for wanting to
separate science and application once one has met the above
prerequisites: (1) That applied interests increase bias and
distortion in the scientific stage, (2) that the technical expert's values are not properly in tune with those of the consumer of technical knowledge or (3) even though there is a
proper balance between the values of the expert and the layman
one rejects the expert's values. Weber held all three of these
reasons. First, great emphasis is placed on the Truth-value of
the scientific research; one can move willy-nilly to isolate it
from possible bias and distortion which would arise from relatively insignificant application interests. Weber was keenly
and properly dissatisfied with the professional-layman value
relationships and this led him to reject application interests
altogether.

There is clear evidence that Weber criticizes his scientific colleagues for two major errors in handling values at the
application stage. The first arises from the tendency of the
scientist to incorporate his own values into policy recommendations to his clients. In applied and clinical science this is
likely to happen when the scientist is in a relatively high-
status position vis-à-vis his client such as the clinical setting of the medical professional. For this reason we have
labeled this situation the "clinical model." It occurs especially in areas where complex technical problems are at stake
and clients are unable or unwilling to master the technical information which would be required to make decisions themselves.
The patient often expects his physician to prescribe a course
of action for him. The policy analysts often expect military
scientists and physicists to make policy judgments. When the
value system of the patient or the client is disregarded and
courses of action are chosen on the basis of the value system
of the scientific consultant there is an excess of professional
value input.

The opposite error is the total elimination of the value system of the applied scientist. In this situation the scientist hires himself out to any and all who will pay for his services. He will prove "value-free" scientific information which can be used by the consumer in any manner he pleases. This frequently occurs in trivial cases such as when an engineer will build any bridge the purchasers order or the chemist will analyze soil samples to order. This situation where there is a minimum of scientist value system incorporated into the decision-making we call the "engineering model." The engineering of napalm manufacture or a supersonic transport plane or perhaps even a trip to the moon for any and all who will pay for it may be examples of the application of science without sufficient inputs from the value system of the scientist especially when he claims that he is performing in his scientific role in a value-free manner.

In his early essays Weber is critical of his colleagues in the *Verein* and their willingness to serve the political interests of the State:

> The Association was dealing with governmental problems (such as the organization of trade unions, taxation, and municipal government and administration), by finding methods of dealing with them that were administratively viable. Which meant making itself useful to Bismarck, the Kaiser, and the German bureaucracy.[24]

Especially in the early years (1904-1905), Weber clearly felt that these men were selling their independence as scientists. They were becoming engineers legitimating social policies without evaluating the policies they were supporting.

In the later essays ("The Meaning of 'Ethical Neutrality'" and "Science as a Vocation") Weber's concern for improper professional-layman value relations shifts to what we have called the clinical model. Scientists are mixing their technical expertise with expertise in values. They are assuming, and the public is granting them, a "generalization of expertise." This is seen particularly in the pattern of professors expounding their personal values in the classroom where there is no opportunity for debate and refutation.[25]

So Weber has encountered firsthand two difficulties with the technical expert becoming involved in the application stage. Even if Weber were not concerned about the relation of the professional's values to those of the layman there is a third reason Weber may have spoken so forcefully in defense of the separation of the scientific stage. Even if Weber could overcome the problem of bias and distortion from application interests and even if he could obtain a proper professional-lay value relationship from his colleagues in the *Verein*, it seems likely that Weber would have been unhappy with their value inputs simply because he disagreed with their value positions. Simey has argued convincingly that there is good evidence for this.[26] He claims:

> The substance of Weber's complaint against the Association, when examined with due care, therefore, amounted to a charge that the values of its leading members such as Schmoller were untenable, not that they had stepped out of the bounds of science by concerning themselves in any way with values as such.[27]

We could claim that this is only part of the story. It appears that Weber was also dissatisfied with the professional-lay value relationships (the clinical and engineering models) and he *did* simply value the scientific pursuit of Truth such that he wanted to maximize effort to eliminate bias and distortion which might arise from application interests.

His solution to the problems created by these difficulties was to join the ranks of the Ionians. Along with Protagoras, the Hippocratic scientific writers, the double-truth theorists of the thirteenth century, Luther, Newton, Locke, and A. J. Ayre are history's dichotomizers. Rather than seeking for a satisfactory solution within the range of applied and clinical science the pure scientists sound a retreat. They are acting from the noblest motives. It is a strategic and temporary retreat to protect the supplies and logistics center. The dichotomizers are convinced that only by the strategic protection of the realm of the scientific can the larger battles be won.

In summary the pure scientist position in the value-dispute is characterized by high regard for the value of Truth, great concern for minimizing bias and distortion combined with

tendencies to disregard deviations from the ideal, relative
minimization of method and other choices involving value inputs, proper dissatisfaction with abusive application efforts,
and a willingness to maintain a thorough-going role separation.

THE APPLIED SCIENCE ASSOCIATIONS

The Society for the Study of Social Problems,
an association of pure and applied social scientists, including sociologists, psychologists, anthropologists, social workers, and other specialists, who are concerned with the following objectives: (1) advancement of the study of social
problems; (2) application of social science research to the formulation of social policies; (3)
improvement of the opportunities and...

The applied scientists represent a complex, intermediate
category between the pure scientists and the radicals. They
have much in common with earlier groups such as the American
Philosophical Society and the American Academy of Arts and Sciences and the Verein für Sozialpolitik. They show the same
missionary zeal in the propagation of knowledge for the solving
of problems. They, in contrast to the pure science associations, realize the complexity of the interactions between science and values. They are different, however. They are professionals (most are members of the pure science associations
of their professions) in revolt against excessive dichotomization of science and values. The applied science associations
arose in response to dissatisfaction with the complete separation of science and application seen in the pure science associations. They generally emerged around the 1940's and 1950's.
The Society for the Psychological Study of Social Issues is an
example, as is its sociological correlate, The Society for the
Study of Social Problems.[28] The Society for Applied Anthropology was organized in 1941 in order to promote scientific investigation of the principles controlling the relations of human
beings to one another (the pure-scientific component) and the
encouragement of the wide application of these principles to
practical problems (the practical vectorial component).

Among the clinically oriented applied natural sciences
there are groups dating from this period including the American

Federation for Clinical Research (1940), the Association of
Clinical Scientists (1949), the Society for Social Responsibility in Science (1949), and, somewhat later, the Academy of Applied Science (1962). The medical sciences also contributed
several of these essentially liberal organizations: Physicians
Forum (1943), the Group for the Advancement of Psychiatry
(1946), and the Association for Applied Psychiatry (1952).

The applied science associations reflect a deep, but
healthy internal conflict and ambiguity about the possibility
of a separation of the scientist and citizen roles. The *Verein
für Sozialpolitik* had as its purpose:

> "supporting the prosperous development" of indus-
> try, "stimulating timely, well-considered state
> intervention to protect the just interests of all
> participants" in the economy, and helping to ac-
> complish "the supreme tasks of our time and our
> nation."[29]

Knapp, in a letter to Schmoller, proposed that in order to
overcome the controversies that had been plaguing the association it "should concentrate on practical issues."[30] The first
two aims of the Society for the Study of Social Problems are
"(1) advancement of the study of social problems; and (2) application of social science research to the formulation of social policy."[31] The statement of purpose of the Society for
the Psychological Study of Social Issues states that "the Society seeks to bring theory and practice into focus on human
problems of the group, the community, and the nation as well as
the increasingly important ones that have no national boundar-
ies."

On the other hand, the applied science associations are
firmly committed to professional integrity and are reluctant to
abandon the scientific role. Daniel Katz, in a study of the
membership of SPSSI concludes:

> The dual role of scientist and citizen may create
> conflict for some, but the great majority of our
> members want both functions retained by SPSSI.[32]

Here we see that the role separation is maintained, but
both roles are at least partially subsumed under the goals of
the professional society. One measure of this role conflict is

the heated debates over whether the society should take stands
on political and public issues. The conflict within SPSSI is
clear. In Katz's study 38 percent of the membership responding indicated that SPSSI should exercise "direct attempts to
influence social action through public stands on social issues"
a great deal.[33] In comparison, 87 percent held that the organization should function in "encouragement and conduct of research on important social issues" a great deal. They are
clearly separating social science and social policy and yet expressing some interest in social policy as well as being clearly committed to focusing their social science on "important social issues." Etzioni, in a recent statement which resembles
the applied science position of reluctant ambiguity presented
here, states that:

> ....as a general rule, a professional association
> ought *not* to comment on public affairs.

but under certain circumstances when "the matter clearly concerns sociological expertise" among other qualifications, and

> if the macroscopic effects of an issue are of
> such magnitude that a *crisis* is reached in the
> sense that basic needs or values *of the society*
> are undermined, the sociological ethic, as I see
> it, makes public comment not simply important,
> but mandatory.[34]

A sociological correlate of this ambiguity about role
separation is the applied science society's ambiguity about
membership qualification. In general, they have a less restrictive policy than the pure science associations. They will
usually accept members who apply, including those clearly in
policy and application fields such as government service and
social work, but they encourage membership from within those
qualified through earned doctorates in the field. As a rule
members will also retain membership in the pure science society.[35]

These factors of role separation and membership criteria
will be seen to be closely related to the associations' handling of the value factors, just as was the case of the pure
science societies. The applied scientist would, of course,
agree with the pure scientist, that values are necessary inputs

in the selection of research topics, but he would tend to differ on the relative weighting of the basic values themselves.
Speaking in very general terms, the applied scientist would not
reject the value of truth or knowledge, even "Truth for Truth's
sake," but would place relatively greater emphasis on the
values of human betterment and moral responsibility in the
sense of using his scientific skills to contribute to solving
social problems. His position is very plausible if one affirms
a pluralistic theory of value. If there are several basic
values in the Aristotelian tradition of G. E. Moore, W. D.
Ross, and most other philosophers of value, one may maximize
utility (goods) by selecting from among the many pursuits of
truth, all of which are intrinsically valuable, those pursuits
which also serve other values including moral responsibility
and human betterment. If you can solve some problems while
pursuing truth why not do so?

There is an even stronger version of this argument. When
other values are placed on a par with or elevated above the
value of truth per se, an even greater moral burden is placed
upon the "pre-scientific" selection of areas of study. Truth,
for the applied scientist, never exists in a vacuum. It is always truth for some potential application. As long as other
values such as happiness and moral responsibility are factors
in this decision, the scientist is confronted with an obligation to consider the potential uses of his investigation in
making such a decision. The Society for Social Responsibility
in Science incorporating this principle announces that its purpose is

> to induce, by education and example, individual
> scientists and engineers to recognize a personal
> responsibility for the anticipated consequences
> to society of their work and the exercise of
> their profession always for the benefit of
> humanity.

While two potential investigations may be of similar value
in advancing knowledge, one may have anticipated uses which are
so threatening that the total value is greatly diminished while
another may have more positive anticipated uses increasing
greatly the value of the project.

Moving to the scientific stage value inputs, the applied scientist would have no difficulties with the scientific study of values and value feedback.[36] He is just as concerned about eliminating bias and distortion as is the pure scientist. Schmoller, commenting on Weber's challenge to the *Verein* said:

> I don't see anything difficult in emphasizing the necessity for purely objective observations. I only see at the ultimate end of this kind of understanding which we arrive at through the social sciences, the appraisal of what is known from the point of view of the whole, of which it is a part.[37]

The applied scientists differ from their pure scientist counterparts, however, in their willingness to really come to terms with the deviations from the ideal of eliminating bias and distortion. Kelman, in an address to the Society for Applied Anthropology, devotes considerable attention to "The Paucity of Independent and International Research."[38] The applied scientists' awareness of the importance of values in choices regarding theory, methodology, and data recording and reporting is what we would term "undeveloped." There is emerging among applied scientists a "left-wing" who perhaps fall into the narrow crevice between the liberals of the applied science societies and the radicals. Such men as Gouldner, Horowitz, Kelman, and perhaps even Becker, in spite of his bitter debate with Gouldner, show great sensitivity to the necessity of value inputs into method and other choices at the scientific stage.[39] This awareness together with their realistically dealing with short-comings in the ideal of eliminating bias and distortion has led to great concern with taking value inputs into account and controlling for their necessary presence.[40] On the other hand, the applied science associations also include members who are more directly interested in industrial and administrative uses of social science who tend to be less aware of this need.

We have commented on the applied scientists' relative interest in social responsibility in comparison with the pure scientists' pursuit of Truth. This is related to a final value factor of the scientific stage, moral evaluation of the research. While the societies, themselves, have not always been effective in ethical criticism of research,[41] individual members of the applied science societies have led the battle for moral evaluation of research from the two perspectives we identified, ethical examination of the research procedures themselves and reflection on the potential uses of the research. This is the logical consequence of their pluralistic value theory whereby truth value is constantly competing with moral and social values.[42]

In the application stage the applied scientists show the ambiguity predictable from their ambiguity about the possibility of role separation. We have already pointed to differences within the societies' memberships which imply differences in the handling of value inputs in the application stage. Some applied scientists, interested in industrial and administrative use of social science, have tendencies toward becoming social engineers which in its extreme form can lead to attempts to "bracket" one's personal values in a value-free manner and a corresponding insensitivity to the social implications of their technological contributions. The Hawthorne works study is an example of this type of social engineering.

Others, such as Gouldner in his Presidential Address to the Society for the Study of Social Problems, attacks those who have:

> used the value-free postulate as an excuse for
> pursuing their private impulses to the neglect
> of their public responsibilities and who, far
> from becoming morally sensitive, become morally
> jaded.[43]

The applied science societies have also showed willingness to criticize the faults of our clinical model, although in other cases they have been guilty of just such practices as in the case of the *Verein's* social policy makers. Burgess, in his Address to the SSSP, is aware of the error of the excess professional value inputs in the clinical model:

> Research on values, however, does not qualify the
> sociologist to become the dictator of values to a
> society. His role is limited to presenting his
> findings, analyzing the issues, pointing out trends,
> and indicating the probable consequences of dif-
> ferent courses of action.[44]

In summary, the applied scientist shows an ambiguity in his handling of the value inputs in the application stage. On the one hand he retains a longing for the old ideal of value-freedom and role separation. On the other hand he, upon occasion, realizes the impossibility and ethical dangers of that move and advocates a balanced use of values in the application of his scientific knowledge avoiding the dangers of the engineering and clinical models.

THE RADICAL ASSOCIATIONS

> The assembly here tonight is a kind of a lie. It is not a coming together of those who study and know, or promote study and knowledge of, social reality. It is a conclave of high and low priests, scribes, intellectual valets, and their innocent victims, engaged in the mutual affirmation of a falsehood, in common consecration of a myth.
>
> Martin Nicolaus, "Remarks at ASA Convention (1968)"[45]

A new type of professional social science group, the radicals, has emerged in the social crisis of the 1960's and early 1970's. It remains to be seen how durable they will be. In contrast to the applied social scientists who reluctantly and cautiously combined the roles of scientist and citizen, the life-blood of the radicals' program is the rejection of any possibility of role separation. The New York *Times* reported on the radical challenge to the September, 1969, meetings of the American Sociological Association saying that the center of the dispute was the question of the role of the sociologist.[46] The basic pattern of the radical caucuses is to demand that the associations, as institutional bodies, take positions on public, social issues. This contrasts with the great hesitancy of the applied social science societies to take such stands. Young radicals at the 1969 ASA meetings wore black arm bands acknowledging the death of Ho Chi Minh;[47] the Psychologists for Democratic Action asked the 1969 APA meeting to support amnesty for all Black Panthers including Eldridge Cleaver and to send relief money to Cuba for hurricane victims;[48] the radical caucus of the American Historical Association demanded that the

Association denounce the war in Viet Nam and called for a "re-evaluation of the assumptions of American foreign policy."[49]

This radical rejection of role separation has the predictable correlate in membership criteria. The radical group, Concerned Asian Scholars, will accept anyone expressing an interest in Asian affairs; the Medical Committee on Human Rights has a similar policy for those interested in social aspects of health, the Eastern Union of Radical Sociologists' membership form includes the line where professional status is indicated "DK;NA____." This openness in membership criteria combined with the natural interests of the group gives rise to an interesting contrast with the applied and pure scientists. Whereas the pure scientists are concerned with social problems in the very long run at best, and the applied scientists are interested primarily on humanitarian or business grounds, the radicals tend to have direct, firsthand experience of the problems about which they are concerned. In most of these groups the overwhelming majority of the members represent relatively low status, oppressed, or minority groups. This is true for the Black Psychologists' Association, the Black Student Psychologists' Association, Black Sociologists, and the organization for women's liberation among the delegates to the ASA meetings. Students, who now consider themselves an oppressed, low-status group, and who were susceptible to the immediate threats of the draft and the war, play a leading role in virtually all the other radical groups including the Sociology Liberation Movement and its successors, the Eastern and Western Unions of Radical Sociologists, the radical caucus in the American Historical Association, Concerned Asian Scholars, Psychologists for Social Action, and the Psychologists for a Democratic Society.

The radicals' handling of the various value factors in the scientific enterprise is closely related to their views on role separation. They place strong emphasis on the pre-scientific selection of topics in accord with their basic values. In their relative weighing of basic values they stand at the opposite extreme from the pure scientist. They ask with Pilate and modern anti-metaphysical philosophers, "What is Truth?" For

the radical, knowledge and the scientific enterprise is viewed
primarily instrumentally, for its value in solving social problems. "Truth for Truth's sake" becomes a derogatory slogan.
The radical chides the establishment scientist for finding "sociologically interesting" those studies which benefit the upper
classes and ruling elites. In the words of Nicolaus:

> Eyes down, to study the activities of the lower
> classes, of the *subject* population--those activ-
> ities which created problems for the smooth
> exercise of governmental hegemony.[50]

The radical also criticizes the establishment scientist
for being scared off by the risks, political and otherwise,
from engaging in socially relevant research. This view is seen
in the Concerned Asian Scholar's critique of the Association
for Asian Studies for limiting its work to relatively sterile,
safe subjects following the attacks on the AAS's predecessor,
the Institute of Pacific Relations.[51]

The 1969 and 1970 meetings of the American Association for
the Advancement of Science were confronted with challenges by a
group calling itself Scientists and Engineers for Social and
Political Action (SESPA). It also uses the alternate name
"Science for the People."[52] This "non-organization," as they
call themselves, was generated in January of 1969. Its birth
pangs were heard at the meetings of the American Physical Society that month. By December they were prepared for major
actions at the Bostom meetings of the AAAS. The major theme of
their confrontations with the AAAS has been the accusation of
what they consider to be hypocrisy in the promotion of scientists' personal and economic interests in the name of the pursuit of truth and scientific value-free objectivity.[53] Like
the applied scientists, but in a much more vigorous and radical
fashion, they attacked the notion that any scientific activity
can be undertaken without responsibility for its potential
uses. They, in their own words:

> chastized the scientific establishment for un-
> critically creating knowledge, technology, and
> hardware which promoted military and corporate
> interests through the impoverishment and oppression
> of people here in America and around the world.

> We are here in Chicago to continue that struggle,
> and to drive home the point that scientific work
> has become inevitably political.[54]

This brings us to the second stage, that of the scientific enterprise per se. We find that the radical is almost obsessively committed to making the point that method and other choices must be present in any so-called scientific study. The *Insurgent Sociologist* attacks the sociological power elite's value inputs into choices of concepts and methods and into their choices of what is significant for publication:

> The task of the sociological power elite that
> controls the ASA, the major university depart-
> ments, the allocations of research funds, and
> the acceptance of manuscripts by the major
> publishers, is to define sociology and social
> reality, to mutually affirm that definition,
> and to enforce their definitions on other
> sociologists, as well as subject groups....
> Radical sociologists, in the SLM are challeng-
> ing the value premises, concepts, methodology,
> and conclusions of establishment sociology.[55]

It is clear, however, that they are not doing this in the name of value-freedom. The Eastern Union of Radical Sociologists has called for the development of a "radical methodology."[56]

At times the radical integration of the scientific and the moral has gone even beyond this observation that methodology and other decisions within the scientific operation are value dependent. The radical is sensitive to the utter collapse of any distinction between the evaluative and the scientific category called sinful or evil behavior. While the pure scientist, Talcott Parsons, has maintained that the differentiation of types of deviance is crucial to the scientific enterprise,[57] radical thinkers such as Thomas Szasz[58] and Morton Schatzman challenge the over-dichotomization of the scientific and the moral. Schatzman says:

> Psychiatric practice in the mental hospital has
> been a *moral* tactic, cloaked with the dignity of
> scientific truth.[59]

Their vocal criticism of ignoring value inputs in method and other choices has led them to place relatively little emphasis on value inputs in the form of bias and distortion in the use of selected methods and in the recording and reporting of observations. It is clear, however, that they are thoroughly convinced that the scientist is far from achieving the ideal of value-freedom in this sphere. In fact they are so thoroughly committed to the pervasiveness of the ideological distortion of both method choices and objective execution once decisions are made that one cannot help but fear that the radicals may completely lose sight of the validity and significance of the *goal* of eliminating bias and distortion from these executions.

The radicals stand with the applied scientists in offering a vigorous ethical critique of research which is deceptive, without informed consent, physically or psychologically dangerous, dehumanizing, or otherwise ethically questionable in and of itself. The radicals' complete rejection of role separation, however, leads them, as in the case of taking stands on political issues, to a greater willingness to deal institutionally with these ethical issues. They also offer vocal insistence upon the feedback loop from application to moral evaluation of the scientific enterprise. This leads us to the third or application stage.

We have seen that Weber appeared to have three motives for affirming value-freedom: (1) the danger of bias and distortion from application interests, (2) dissatisfaction from excesses (clinical) and deficiencies (engineering) in the technical expert's value inputs in relationship to the layman's, and (3) direct dissatisfaction with the values held by Schmoller and the members of the *Verein*. The first motive requires relatively high value on scientific knowledge itself and the potential or ideal possibility of value-freedom in the scientific stage. The radicals must reject Weber's move on both counts. They place relatively high value in the instrumental uses of scientific knowledge in the application stage and relatively low value on the knowledge itself. Their strong emphasis on the necessity of value-inputs from method and other choices as well as moral evaluation of the process excludes value-freedom even as an ideal.

Weber's second motive is shared by the radicals. They are intensely concerned about what we have termed excesses and

deficiencies in technical expert value inputs. Their most out-
spoken criticism is directed toward the moral escapism of the
extreme forms of our engineering model. Kagan criticizes the
failure of the Association of Asian Scholars for eschewing involvement in public activities so that "The scholar's public
service role was re-defined, re-oriented, from one of instruction at large to that of the expert and social technician."[60]
Two of the resolutions presented by the Eastern Union of Sociologists to the 1969 ASA meetings called for condemning "participation of any of its members in the NIMH-funded research
concerning the 'protest-prone' student."[61] But the radicals
are also sensitive to the elitism of the clinical model rejecting the notion that the elite status of the establishment social scientist gives special weight to his value premises or
conclusions.[62] In contrast to Weber, however, the escape route
behind the wall of value-free science is closed because of the
basic value of solving social problems and the impossibility of
a value-free ideal at the scientific stage.

This leaves them groping for some new model of professional-lay relations which relates the professional to the application stage of his work. The retreat to pure science is
blocked. The escape route of the applied scientists must maintain the link of their scientific work to the application
stage. They do so by trying to balance the professional's
value inputs avoiding the excesses of the clinical model and
the deficiencies of the engineering model. This can become
romanticized and platitudinous. The radicals, in contrast, are
sensitive to the requirements of substructural equality which
are necessary if there is to be any attempt to balance the
professional-lay value inputs. This leaves them in the uncom-
fortable position of flatly rejecting the value-free ideal and
even running the risk of eclipsing it by their nearly total de
facto rejection of role separation, and at the same time finding two of the application stage models unacceptable while the
middle position is not feasible without radical social trans-
formation.

This completes our analysis of the major positions that
professional groups have taken with regard to these value

factors. Each alternative is seen to provide major contributions to the dispute and to have made or run the risk of making serious errors. We are convinced, however, that only by becoming aware of the complexities and interactions of the multiplicity of value factors involved in the great *Werturteilsstreit* will the issues and the solutions emerge.

NOTES

CHAPTER I

[1]Several accounts of the emergence of modern scientific
societies have been helpful in preparing this discussion. See
Martha Ornstein, *The Role of Scientific Societies in the
Seventeenth Century* (Chicago: University of Chicago Press,
1938); Abraham Wolf (ed.), *A History of Science, Technology
and Philosophy in the 16th and 17th Centuries* (New York:
Harper, 1959); and Ralph S. Bates, *Scientific Societies in the
United States*, 3rd ed. (Cambridge, Mass.: The Massachusetts
Institute of Technology Press, 1965).

[2]Benjamin Franklin, *Autobiography*, cited in Bates, p. 5.

[3]American Philosophical Society Proceedings, III (1843)
9, cited in Bates, *Scientific Societies*, p. 6.

[4]Bates, *Scientific Societies*, pp. 28-30.

[5]Deutsche Gesellschaft für Soziologie. Verhandlungen des
Ersten Deutschen Soziologentages. Tübingen: Mohr, 1911, v,
cited in Rolf Dahrendorf, "Values and Social Science," *Essays
in the Theory of Society* (Stanford, California: Stanford University, 1968), p. 2.

[6]Max Weber, "The Meaning of 'Ethical Neutrality' in
Sociology and Economics," in *The Methodology of the Social Sciences* (New York: The Free Press, 1949), p. 11.

[7]The following historical account is pieced together from
the history of the Verein für Sozialpolitik by Franz Boese,
Geschichte des Vereins für Sozialpolitik, 1872-1939 (Berlin:
Duncker und Humblot, 1939); also, Ralf Dahrendorf, "Values and
Social Science"; T. S. Simey, "Max Weber: Man of Affairs or
Theoretical Sociologist," *Sociological Review*, 14 (No. 1966),
303-328; and Eduard Baumgarten, *Max Weber, Work and Person*
(Tübingen: Mohr, 1964). Boese was secretary of the Verein un-
til 1936 when it dissolved and writes from the Schmoller per-
spective.

[8]The four most significant of Weber's papers pertaining
to the value-dispute are, "'Objectivity' in Social Science and
Social Policy" (1904), "The Logic of the Cultural Sciences
(1905), "The Meaning of 'Ethical Neutrality' in Sociology and
Economics" (1917), all translated and reprinted in *The Methodology of the Social Sciences* (New York: The Free Press, 1949)
and "Science as a Vocation," in *From Max Weber: Essays in Sociology*, ed. by Hans Gerth and C. Wright Mills (New York: Oxford University Press, 1958), pp. 129-56.

[9]Dahrendorf, "Values and Social Science," p. 3.

[10]Simey, "Max Weber," p. 307; Dahrendorf, "Values and Social Science," p. 1.

41

[11]Max Weber, "The Meaning of 'Ethical Neutrality' in
Sociology and Economics," in *The Methodology of the Social
Sciences* (New York: The Free Press, 1949), p. 60.

[12]Deutsche Gesellschaft für Soziologie Verhandlungen des
Ersten Deutschen Soziologentages (Tübingen: Mohr, 1911) V,
cited in Dahrendorf, "Values and Social Science," p. 2.

[13]Deutsche Gesellschaft für Soziologie Verhandlungen des
Zweiten Deutschen Soziologentages (Tübingen: Mohr, 1913), p.
78, cited in Dahrendorf, "Values and Social Science," p. 3.

[14]See "The American Sociological Society," in *Papers and
Proceedings Annual Meeting*, I (1906), pp. 1-2; Lester F. Ward,
"The Establishment of Sociology," *Papers and Proceedings,
Annual Meeting*, I (1906), p. 309; and R. J. Halliday, "The
Sociological Movement, The Sociological Society, and the Gene-
sis of Academic Sociology in Britain," *Sociological Review*, XVII
(1968), 377-98.

[15]Wilse B. Webb, "The Organization of Psychologists, Their
Training and Their Employment," in *The Profession of Psychology*
(New York: Holt, Rinehart, and Winston, 1968), p. 34.

[16]Weber, "Science as a Vocation," p. 145; also see "The
Meaning of 'Ethical Neutrality,'" p. 5.

[17]Read Bain, "Science, Values, and Sociology," *American
Sociological Review*, IV (August, 1937), 562-63.

[18]Weber, "The Meaning of 'Ethical Neutrality,'" p. 21.
Also see Bain, "Science, Values, and Sociology," p. 562; Weber,
"The Logic of the Cultural Sciences," p. 169.

[19]Weber, "The Meaning of 'Ethical Neutrality,'" p. 11.

[20]Simey, "Max Weber," p. 326, note 27.

[21]Weber, "The Meaning of 'Ethical Neutrality,'" p. 11.

[22]Ward, "The Establishment of Sociology," p. 3.

[23]The second fallacy of the ideal type is to behave as if
the ideal could be reached, even ideally. Bain implies this
fallacy by suggesting that if the scientist can only stick to
his scientific methodology, then he will achieve value-free
objectivity. He says that the scientist's "methodology has
been developed so as to minimize the distortions of personal,
private, limited experience. If this methodology is violated,
experience shows that his observation, classification, hypotheses, manipulations, and conclusions fail of the impersonal,
nonmoral objectivity which is the methodological goal of
natural science." Bain, "Science, Values, and Sociology," p.
562.

[24]Simey, "Max Weber," p. 319.

[25] Weber, "The Meaning of 'Ethical Neutrality'," p. 7; also "Science as a Vocation," p. 145.

[26] Simey, "Max Weber," pp. 326, 317, 318, 322.

[27] Simey, "Max Weber," p. 322.

[28] See Ernest W. Burgess, "The Aims of the Society for the Study of Social Problems," *Social Problems*, I (1953), pp. 2-3.

[29] Dahrendorf, "Values and Social Science," p. 3.

[30] Simey, "Max Weber," p. 311.

[31] The SSSP statement of objectives has changed slightly through the years of its existence. This list was taken from the frontispiece in *Social Problems*, I (1953).

[32] Daniel Katz, "Organizational Effectiveness and Change; An Evaluation of SPSSI by Members and Former Members," *The Journal of Social Issues*, supplement series, number 11, (1958), p. 8.

[33] Katz, "Organizational Effectiveness and Change," p. 7.

[34] Amitai Etzioni, "On Public Affairs Statements of Professional Associations," *The American Sociologist*, III (Nov. 1968), pp. 279-80.

[35] The same was true, but in reverse, in the German dispute. The pure scientists, being the younger, reacting group, retained their membership in the *Verein*.

[36] See Ernest W. Burgess, "Values and Sociological Research," *Social Problems*, I (1953), pp. 16-20, especially 17, where in the Presidential Address to the Society for the Study of Social Problems, he defends not only the possibility, but also the necessity of scientific study of values.

[37] Cited in Simey, "Max Weber," p. 311.

[38] Herbert C. Kelman, *A Time to Speak* (San Francisco: Jossey-Bass, Inc., 1968), p. 92.

[39] See Howard Becker, "Whose Side Are We On?" *Social Problems*, XIV (Winter, 1967), 239-47, where in a Presidental Address to the Society for the Study of Social Problems, he comes squarely to terms with the necessity for these value choices, and compare this with Alvin W. Gouldner's critique from an even more radical perspective in "The Sociologist as Partisan: Sociology and the Welfare State," *The American Sociologist*, 2 (May, 1968), 103-16. This should be contrasted with Gouldner's earlier Presidential Address to the Society for the Study of Social Problems, "Anti-Minotaur: The Myth of Value-Free Sociology," in *Sociology on Trial*, ed. by Maurice Stein and Arthur Vidich, (Englewood Cliffs, N.J.: Prentice-Hall, Inc., 1963),

pp. 35-52, which was a major contribution to the contemporary phase of the value-dispute, but which develops this particular aspect of the critique less fully.

[40]See Kelman, *A Time to Speak*, pp. 59, 72-3.

[41]See Leonard D. Cain, Jr., "The AMA and the Gerontologists: Uses and Abuses of 'A Profile of the Aging: USA'," in *Ethics, Politics, and Social Research*, ed. by Gideon Sjoberg (Cambridge, Mass.: Schenkman Publishing Company, Inc., 1967), pp. 78-114, especially 103-04.

[42]Kelman, *A Time to Speak*, pp. 208-25, for an example of the first type. See *The Rise and Fall of Project Camelot*, ed. by Irving Horowitz, (Cambridge: The Massachusetts Institute of Technology Press, 1967), for an example of the second type.

[43]Gouldner, "Anti-Minotaur: The Myth of Value-Free Sociology," p. 42.

[44]Burgess, "Values and Sociological Research," p. 20.

[45]Martin Nicolaus, "Remarks at ASA Convention," *The American Sociologist*, IV (May, 1969), p. 155.

[46]"Radicals Chide 'Uptight' Sociologists on the Coast," New York *Times*, September 6, 1969, p. 25.

[47]*Ibid.*

[48]"Blacks Supported by Psychologists," New York *Times*, September 3, 1969, p. 34.

[49]"Leftist Historians," Chicago *Tribune*, January 2, 1970, p. 20.

[50]Nicolaus, "Remarks at ASA Convention," p. 155.

[51]Richard Kagan, "McCarran's Legacy: The Association for Asian Studies," *Bulletin of Concerned Asian Scholars*, IV (May, 1969), p. 19.

[52]Herb Fox, "SESPA: A History," *Science for the People*, II, No. 4 (December, 1970), pp. 2-3.

[53]"A History of the AAAS or You Been a Good Ole Wagon, But You Done Broke Down," *Science for the People*, II, No. 4 (December, 1970), pp. 15-16.

[54]People's Science Collective, New University Conference, "Science For the People," mimeographed and distributed at the AAAS meetings in Chicago, December, 1970.

[55]*The Insurgent Sociologist: Counter-Convention Call*, Berkeley, California: *Insurgent Sociologist*, (1969), p. 3.

[56]"Eastern Union of Radical Sociologists," open letter to colleagues, July, 1969, p. 3.

[57]Talcott Parsons, "Definitions of Health and Illness in the Light of American Values and Social Structure," in E. Gartley Jaco, (ed.), *Patients, Physicians and Illness* (New York: The Free Press, 1958), pp. 165-87.

[58]Thomas Szasz, *The Myth of Mental Illness* (New York: Harper, 1961).

[59]Morton Schatzman, "Madness and Morals," in *Radical Therapist*, I, No. 4 (October-November, 1970), p. 11.

[60]Kagan, "McCarran's Legacy," p. 70.

[61]*The Insurgent Sociologist*, p. 41.

[62]*The Insurgent Sociologist*, p. 2.

CHAPTER II

TOWARD A UNIFIED THEORY OF A MEDICAL ACTION SYSTEM

In the introductory section we have provided a brief syn-
opsis of history's ongoing battle over the relationship of the
scientific and technological enterprise to systems of meaning
and evaluation. In the next three chapters we shall attempt a
systematic theoretical formulation of this relationship. The
present chapter will be devoted to the initial construction of
a model of a unified theory of action in the scientific context focusing on the place of values in that action system.
The next chapter will focus more narrowly on the evaluation
component in that system, relating ethical to other types of
evaluation, values to more generalized systems of value orientation, and ultimate values (which have a high level of generality) to what we shall call the cultural value complex (which
functions at a much more specific level). In the last chapter
of our theoretical formulation we shall shift our perspective
from one of attempting to place values within the larger system
of action to a more dynamic analysis of the many points in the
process of scientific and technological activity where values
may be involved.

One of the points that we shall make during the course of
this analysis is that any methodology or theoretical construction used for scientific and technological activity necessarily
carries with it certain value assumptions. This applies, no
less, to our own theoretical construction. In the present
chapter we shall offer an action system analysis heavily dependent upon Parsonian categories and methodology. It is a commonly heard charge that Parsonian theory has a "conservative"
bias. While there is a certain legitimacy in this claim, especially as the theory has been used by many of the better known
Parsonians, the charge is highly over-simplified. When making
such a claim one must be careful to separate biases inherent in
the methodology itself from those of the users of the methodology. We shall point out during the course of the chapter several instances where analysts of the medical action system have

incorporated "conservative" assumptions into their analysis,
but we shall suggest that many of these can be corrected by
minor localized therapeutic procedures on the analysis itself
without the radical systemic surgery which is often prescribed.

On the other hand it is justifiable to accuse action system theory of orienting analysis to static phenomena with relatively little attention given to the dynamic aspects of process, change, development, and system revolution, which are en-
demic in conflict and cybernetic theories. In the final chapter of the theoretical construction we shall shift our methodology in order to look at the many points in the scientific and
technological process where, for better or worse, values may be
incorporated. Here we shall construct a cybernetic model and
propose alternatives for the professional-lay relationship
which are rooted in rather different theoretical methods.[1]

The task of the present chapter is to make an initial attempt to construct a unified theoretical model for the scientific and technological enterprise and to locate the points in
the system where values play a part. While we are interested
in a model for science and technology generally we have decided
to build our construction from the bag of tools which are
available from the theorists who have worked in medical sociology. We have done this for several reasons. This is a very
complex enterprise and to incorporate the literature from all
aspects of science and technology would be inevitably confusing
as well as being beyond the limits of the author's ability. By
building our model with specific reference to the theoretical
tools of the medical sociologists we are working with a compre-
hensible and consistent body of literature. Nevertheless we
would maintain that the model we construct from these pieces is
capable of universalization to the scientific and technological
action system more generally. We shall be using medicine as a
type-case for a much broader category of lay-professional relationships.

The place of the social and cultural sciences in the field
of medicine is becoming firmly established. During the course
of the last few decades empirical verification of the importance of socio-cultural factors in the etiology, diagnosis, and

treatment of disease and the promotion of health has been complemented by a number of theoretical constructions which attempt to indicate the social element in medical action. The seminal contribution by L. J. Henderson entitled "Physician and Patient as a Social System" is only the first in a series of important, if fragmentary, theoretical contributions to the sociology of medicine.[2] Bloom[3] and Wilson[4] are among those who have been stimulated by his article to modify and expand the conception of the physician-patient relationship as a unit of social interaction.

In his extremely important chapter in *The Social System*, Talcott Parsons[5] has applied his pattern variable schema to the patient-physician relationship. Here he also offered a conception of the "sick role," which has become a major theoretical tool in the sociology of medicine[6] and the professional counterpart to the sick role is his description of the role pattern of the physician.[7] In the mid-fifties important empirical research was done on the significance of the socialization of the medical student.[8] Finally, on a broader plane, several contributions to the sociology of knowledge have provided models for our understanding of decision-making processes.[9]

All of these contributions are elements in the theoretical development of the sociology of medicine. In this chapter we shall make a preliminary attempt to combine these pieces of a theoretical jig-saw puzzle into a unified theory of a medical action system. While the puzzle may not be completely assembled in this effort, we hope to at least construct the border and fit together enough of the pieces so that we have a hint of the completed picture.

A. A PRELIMINARY MODEL OF A MEDICAL ACTION SYSTEM

One thinks first of the relationship of the patient to the physician as one which is designed to execute a specific problem-solving task. A set of symptoms indicates a condition, generally of an organic nature, for which an expert in the application of medical science must be consulted. The sociologically alert, however, will be aware that this generates a system of social interaction which is not totally instrumental.

Henderson was a physiologist and a physician who was strongly influenced by the work of Willard Gibbs on the equilibrium of chemical substances in the body, particularly in the blood. Gibbs conceptualized substances in the material universe as "physico-chemical systems." Henderson compared Gibbs' physiological conception of a "system" to the Italian sociologist, Pareto's, description of a generalized *social* system.[10] Applying this to the medical situation, Henderson proposed that a physician and a patient make up a social system.

Henderson's main contribution in his paper, which was originally presented to students at Harvard Medical School, was to stress the importance of what he called "sentiments" in the relationship between physician and patient. He claimed:

> In any social system the sentiments and the inter-actions of the sentiments are likely to be the most important phenomena....The patient is moved by fears and by many other sentiments, and these, together with reason, are being modified by the doctor's words and phrases, by his manner and expression.[11]

He warned the medical students not to let the patient's sentiments modify their behavior, while at the same time he stressed the importance of real interest in the patient on the part of the physician. The social system described by Henderson is diagrammed in Figure 1.

Figure 1 can be viewed as a minimal system of interaction between two individuals in which there is both instrumental and emotional or expressive interchange. Henderson's conceptualization has carried us a long way from the naive view of medicine which tends to overlook the human factors in the interaction. Our Figure 1 is meant to convey a preliminary and isolated model of interaction not dissimilar to the first model proposed by Samuel W. Bloom.[12] Several modifications are necessary, however, in order to make Henderson's formulation coincide with the discoveries of the rapidly expanding field of sociology of medicine. We shall propose three basic modifications: generalization of the actors in the social system, emphasis on the multi-directional nature of the interchange, and addition of socio-cultural components to the system.

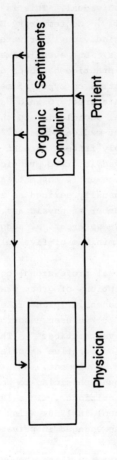

Fig. 1. A Preliminary Model of the Medical Action System

1. *Generalization of the Actors.*

The solo "fee-for-service" physician is the stereotype of
the medical practitioner, at least in the United States. It is
implied in the Henderson discussion of the physician and the
patient. Upon reflection it is clear that the medical practitioner is not always an individual. This is particularly true
when viewed cross-culturally. Contemporary European medicine
does not have the norm of individual, private practice which
exists in the United States. But even in American medical
practice the idea of solo practice has been described as a
myth.[13] Up to date statistics on types of medical practice are
difficult to obtain and interpret. Oswald Hall's work in the
forties alerted the medical sociologist to the growing importance of different types of medical careers.[14] It has been
estimated that approximately fifteen percent of American physicians are currently involved in group practice. This seems
like a fairly small fraction until the matter is probed further. Group practice is usually defined as a formal, legal
association involving a number of physicians. Jordan, in his
volume *The Physician and Group Practice*, suggests that the term
be limited to groups of a minimum of five full-time physicians.[15]

Many formal and informal professional collectivities are
not included in the descriptions of group practices such as
clinics and pre-paid comprehensive plans like the Health Insurance Plan of New York.[16] Freidson describes several "elementary forms of cooperative practice."[17] These include the
small, legal partnership; cooperative association with common
facilities such as offices, equipment, and assisting personnel;
and the employment of a young physician to work in the office
of a successful senior practitioner. In a 1960 study of the
graduates from medical school in 1950, Weiskotten found that
sixty-four percent of those engaged in private practice were
practicing alone.[18]

Even among those practicing alone, however, we cannot con-
ceive of the professional actor as an isolated physician. Hall
has described the system of formal and informal contacts among
colleagues which provides for social interaction on the part of

the professionals.[19] We shall describe the importance of professional collectivities and colleague networks later in this
study. We are here interested in how the individual patient
consulting an individual physician practicing alone nonetheless
interacts with a plurality of professionals.

There are two primary ways in which this may take place:
first, the highly developed referral system, and, second, the
treatment of patients in the hospital complex. In both cases,
although the patient makes contact with practitioners practicing alone, he still is involved in a professional complex of a
plurality of individuals. When it is realized that the paramedical personnel also form part of the medical team, it is
fair to say that in virtually all cases the professional component in the medical action system is supra-individual. Following standard sociological usage, in which the term "actor" may
refer to either an individual or a collectivity, we feel that
it is necessary to generalize the term "physician" by referring
to the "professional actor" in the medical system. This should
be taken as referring to the entire medical team, which in the
limiting case may be the isolated physician.

It seems much closer to reality to view the patient as an
individual. (This is not to say that there is not a strong
social element in health, disease, and medical action. We
shall discuss this below.) There are cases, however, where the
"patient" in some sense is a collectivity. This is so when a
group must be treated by the same professional actor such as in
the hospital ward or in civil or military disaster. It is also
the case when a medical condition arises out of the interaction
of two individuals such as mother and child. We shall substi-
tute the term "lay actor" for patient in order to generalize
the layman's side of the interaction process.

The dominance of the individualized patient-physician relationship as a conceptual tool in medicine and medical sociology is not without its ideological significance. It is consistent with and supportive of the individualistic orientation of
the medical profession. It is in part a defense of the sanc-
tity of the physician's private and personal relationship with
his patient which, so the rhetoric of the American Medical

Association tells us, cannot be violated by intervention from social and political agents. This is an example of the bias which can frequently be incorporated into theoretical formulations even in the seemingly value-free task of abstract description of the relationship of the medical professional to his client. However, this does not mean that the action system analysis which gives rise to the conceptualization of the patient-physician relationship need necessarily be rejected. The generalization of the professional and lay actors, as indicated in Figure 2, maintains the interaction perspective while correcting for the individualistic bias of the more common terminology.

2. *The Multi-directional Nature of the Interchange.*

We have indicated in Figure 1 our interpretation of Henderson's description of the patient-physician interaction. The instrumental action is primarily from the physician (professional actor) to the patient (lay actor) in the form of efforts to cure disease. The expressive action, however, primarily originates from the patient. The physician should be aware of the importance of sentiments, should see to it that they do not interfere with the medical procedure, and above all, "should endeavor to act upon the patient's sentiments according to a well-considered plan."[20] In what to us is one of the insensitivities of Henderson's prophetic paper, he reveals a tendency, at times, to endow his physicians, and the future physicians he was addressing, with superior skill in the art of objectivity. This tendency he shares with Freudians whom he accuses of rationalizations and "quasi-religious enthusiasms."[21] While he "talks reason and good sense" with the students, he warns that these tactics should not be used with patients:

> It is not only to a mob that reason and good sense cannot effectively be talked. A patient sitting in your office, facing you, is rarely in a favorable state of mind to appreciate the precise significance of a logical statement, and it is in general not merely difficult but quite impossible for him to perceive the precise meaning of a train of thought.[22]

This tendency to "talk reason and good sense" when speaking with colleagues, but not while talking with "mobs" or with clients is one of the less savory characteristics of professionalism. It is a characteristic Henderson shares with the cultic physicians who swore to secrecy in the Hippocratic oath. Professionalization takes place by passing on a special gnosis which is too dangerous for the common folk.

The professional actor is characterized by affective neutrality in the ideal-type. There is no doubt that institutional setting and professional socialization provide a degree of control of expressive interchange that is not possible in other social settings, but we must not overlook the exchange of human interaction which is initiated on the professional side. It cannot be denied that expressive interchange is also initiated by the professional actor. It is an oversimplification to say that even ideally they should be eliminated. The suggestion that they should be eliminated in the ideal or, even worse, the overlooking of the deviations from the supposed ideal so that they are not taken into account when they exist in practice is what we, in Chapter IV, shall call the fallacy of the ideal type. This tendency to overlook the non-instrumental component in the professional's component of the interaction system is another example of biases which have crept into medical sociological theory, but the solution, once again, is not the abandoning of the theory, but its modification. We shall discuss "affective neutrality" in more detail below.

Having discussed what analysts of small group dynamics have called the expressive interaction, i.e., that which focuses on the human or social-emotional processes, we shall turn to the instrumental or task-oriented interchange.[23] Our preliminary diagram indicates that the instrumental action is from the professional to the lay actor. However, in order for there to be joint participation in the system, in order to overcome a type of paternalism which is inherent in many professional-lay relationships and the theoretical descriptions of them, it is important that the layman's instrumental contribution be recognized and emphasized. This is true even if the system is "collectively-oriented" (see a fuller discussion below). The cash payment to the professional actor is one type of instrumental exchange. There are other elements, however, which, at least upon occasion, become significant. We feel that opportunities to participate in medical experimentation provide frequently unrecognized instrumental inputs on the part of the patient. The patient-subject is vital to the successful execution of much crucial experimentation. The development of neighborhood medical centers and community controlled health programs in which the medical professionals' instrumental contribution is viewed as a portion of a much larger system of exchange of instrumental goods and services may be a more fundamental way in which the instrumental inputs of (medically) lay actors are brought to an increased level of consciousness. More attention needs to be given to the layman's instrumental contribution to the interchange. Figure 2 indicates the modifications we have proposed thus far for Henderson's analysis of the medical system.

3. *The Addition of Socio-cultural Components.*

We have pointed out that the actors in a medical action system are not always individuals. This was the first introduction of social factors into the analysis. There is another set of social factors, however, which are critical to the understanding of the social actions in the institution of medicine. While in the early stages of sociology of medicine, the main thrust was toward establishing the importance of social factors per se, more recently attention has been given to sorting out different types of social factors. We shall divide our discussion into five main types: the lay actor's socio-cultural context, the lay actor's primary social reference (the family), the professional actor's socio-cultural context, the professional's primary social reference (the profession), and the larger socio-cultural context.

a. *The Lay Actor's Socio-cultural Context.* A basic distinction in the sociological study of medicine has emerged between the study of the social factors in health and disease on the one hand and the social factors in medical care and treatment on the other. The former has been termed the sociology of

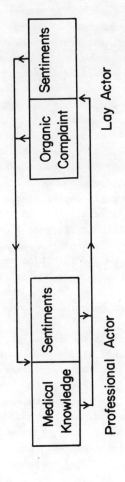

Fig. 2. A Modified Model of the Medical Action System

illness while the latter has been referred to as the sociology of medical care.[24] The physician is frequently more interested in the use of sociology to treat illness, if he has sociological interests at all. This has led to the distinction between sociology *in* medicine and sociology *of* medicine.

Turning first to the sociology of health and illness we shall discuss the socio-cultural factors drawn from the lay actor's subculture. These elements are represented in the right half of Figure 4. Looking at Henderson's 1935 essay from the standpoint of several decades of development in the field of sociology as it relates to medicine, it is quite noticeable that his description of the physician and patient as a social system only begins the movement toward recognition of non-organic factors in medicine. As a physiologist he can be forgiven for limiting his expansion of the medically relevant factors to the patient's "sentiments." To have perceived the importance of this primarily psychological factor as clearly as he did was a great accomplishment. Nevertheless his perspective is still limited. Looking at Figures 1 and 2 once more, it is apparent that the two boxes on the lay actor's side of the diagrams represent two of the four basic subsystems of action, the organic and the psychological. It is imperative if one is to have a total view of the patient and his medical problems that the social and cultural components be brought into consideration.

The lay actor, at least in modern society, represents a unique combination of a number of institutional structures. This unique complex of institutional affiliations mediates in a partial and imperfect way diverse and sometimes contradictory systems of meaning. These meaning systems are partially internalized by the individual actor. If our analysis is to be complete with reference to the lay actor, this unique constellation of social and cultural factors must be included.

This discussion, which reflects contemporary thought in the sociology of knowledge, is applicable to the field of medicine. The social groups in which the lay actor is located are critical for defining behavior which leads to contact, recognition, diagnosis, treatment, and prevention of disease. The

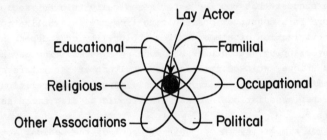

Fig. 3. The Construction of the Lay Actor's Socio-Culture

internalized system of meaning which is an imperfect derivative from the multiple socio-cultural references of the lay actor is critical for the interpretation of symptoms and attachment of meaning to medical conditions. Bloom is aware of the importance of these socio-cultural factors.[25] He first places the patient in the context of his family, which is certainly a primary institutional locus for the patient. He then encloses the family in what he terms the "subcultural reference groups," diagramming the relation with a set of concentric circles.[26]

While this places needed emphasis on the socio-cultural factor, it does not adequately represent the complexity of the pluralism of modern society. One's subcultural reference groups do not completely encompass the family. Following Berger and Luckmann's work in the sociology of knowledge,[27] we would suggest that the lay actor's medically relevant socio-culture is a construction resulting from the internalization or subjectivization of elements from a plurality of independent, but overlapping, structures and meaning systems. The lay actor's unique socio-culture is the resultant of the intersection of familial, occupational, political, educational, religious, and other associational roles. This could be diagrammed as in Figure 3.

For simplicity in our unified model of the medical action system we shall represent the lay actor in the conventional manner as a complex of our subsystems, but it must be made clear that the social and cultural subsystems represent a unique complex of the type we have just described. In Figure 4 we have suggested the further analysis of the social subsystem of the lay actor into possible significant social institutional contexts.

b. *The Lay Actor's Primary Social Reference (The Family)*. Even if the socio-cultural component of the lay actor is the result of the complex interaction, it is still possible to speak of a "primary social reference" for the lay actor. There is little doubt that the family is the primary locus of the lay actor's social construction of medical meaning and the primary determinant of his medically relevant environment. Not only does the family play a major role in determining class status,

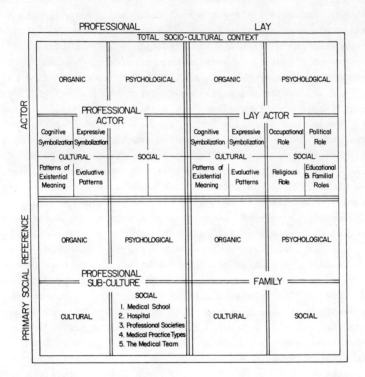

Fig. 4.   A Unified Model of the Medical Action System

residence, and dietary and sanitary habits, it also is the primary transmitter of subcultural value orientations.[28] Modern society is characterized by high functional differentiation of its institutions. The functional task of integration rests primarily with the family along with the educational institutions. Medically relevant socialization, it seems fair to say, takes place principally in the context of the family. It is here that the sick role is learned; it is here that organic processes are assigned meaning and patterns of evaluation and response are developed. We shall thus add to our unified model of medical action the family as the "primary social reference" realizing that this includes the ethnic, subcultural frame of reference into which the family is integrated, and further realizing that the socio-cultural component of the individual lay actor extends beyond the familial context. See Figure 4 where the lay actor's "primary social reference" is included. We have divided this into the four major subsystem components merely to suggest the task of a full sociological analysis of the family which would be necessary to have a full understanding of the primary social reference.

   c. *The Professional Actor's Non-professional Socio-cultural Context.* A similar analysis can be brought to bear on the physician, or in our generalized terminology, the professional actor. He also exists as a human being acting out a complex of roles. It is a fact of the "real world" of medical professionals that there is some disagreement within the profession on just about any case which is presented. It is fair to say that in all cases considered "interesting" from a medical or sociological point of view such disagreement exists. This disagreement is partially a result of uncertainty which is a major factor in the institution of medicine,[29] but nonetheless the positions taken can be seen as arising from two types of sources: the non-professional subculture and differential professional socialization. The elderly, rural, Irish Catholic, female general practitioner (if such a creature exists) can be predicted to take a different position on the use of birth control from the young, Jewish, male specialist working in a large urban research institution.[30]

We shall discuss the structure of medical decision-making below. For now we may simply note that all decision-making is a process of applying value criteria to a set of alternatives. These value criteria are learned, either from one's professional training or from his non-professional associations. The "interesting" alternatives for decision-making involve value choices of the type faced in prescribing therapy for a patient where there are two (or more) alternatives in which one alternative is predictably twice as effective, but twice as risky as the other. Mechanic, in his volume on medical sociology, offers a discussion of this type of problem in which he concludes that "not all doctors develop the same strategies; nor do they opt to take the same kind of risks."[31] He, however, is still more interested in the case where differences occur from the result of imperfect acquaintance with the relevant facts.[32]

In our unified model of a medical action system it will be necessary to represent the professional action as a complex of organic, psychological, social, and cultural factors, just as we did with the lay actor. In this case, also, the social and cultural components are the resultant of a complex interaction of a variety of institutional roles. In Figure 4 this is represented by the analysis of the social factor into several elements as has been done for the lay actor.

We are now at a point where we can emphasize an asymmetry in Figure 2. At first it appears that the instrumental components of the professional and lay actors are parallel in a way in which the sentiment or personality components are. This, however, is not the case. With the lay actor the instrumental component is best understood as a set of organic symptoms (although these must be seen as being interpreted by the cultural apparatus brought to bear by the lay actor). With the professional, however, the primary instrumental component is not the organic, behavioral subsystem of the physician or physician-surrogate. It is the technical, scientific knowledge about the body's organic structure and processes (and about the psyche, to the extent of his psychiatric training) which the professional has learned through the scientific study of medicine. Medicine, in its Western or any other form, is a culturally

developed intellectual discipline involving a culturally trans-
mitted set of cognitive symbols and relations. The behavioral
or organic subsystem of the professional actor is an element in
a total analysis of the medical action system, but it is a
relatively minor factor. The professional's typical patterns
of biological drives such as hunger and sex and other expressions of the behavioral subsystem are of secondary importance.
Below we shall analyze the cultural level symbol systems of the
lay and professional actors into several types of symbolization. For now we shall merely say that the relevant instrumental contribution of the professional actor is a portion of
the cultural subsystem, i.e., that portion which makes use of
the cognitive symbols of the intellectual discipline of medicine. For the lay actor, however, the primary component is in
the behavioral or organic subsystem.

d. *The Professional Actor's Primary Social Reference (Professional Socio-culture)*. For the layman we were able to identify what we called the "primary social reference" in the family. We have claimed that like the layman the professional
must be understood as a complex synthesis of many socio-
cultural factors. It is possible, however, to find a "primary
social reference" for the professional, also. Medicine is a
distinct and recognizable institution. It is this group which
collectively has primary responsibility for the socialization
of future members. It is functionally equivalent to the family
as the "primary social reference" for the professional. The
lower left hand portion of Figure 4 represents the professional
subculture in this manner.

There is one major difference, however, one that is frequently overlooked. The role of practitioner is learned from a
professional subculture which has a high degree of institutionalization. The medical profession is functionally specific,
to use the pattern variable terminology we shall discuss below.
The socialization of the professional is routinized and fairly
clearly defined. Physicians associate in hospital staff meetings and in county medical societies. To a great extent they
read a common set of journals and technical literature. They
have all been through somewhat standardized medical school

curricula, internships and residency programs.[33] The sick role, however, has minimal institutionalization, largely because it is only temporarily legitimated in most cases. The family is a functionally diffuse institution, and its "teaching" of the sick role varies considerably partially as a function of the family's subcultural identification. It is very rare that there exists a formal association of lay medical actors. This does emerge with relatively long illness and continual association of patients such as in a hospital ward where patient interaction has been shown to be very important, but it is the exception rather than the rule.[34]

With the development of third-party payment and group insurance plans there emerges the potential for further development of associations of lay actors. Another source for this development can be seen in the emergence of neighborhood groups organized to effect changes in the health care delivery in their community. Nonetheless at the present, the general absence of such associations represents an important difference between professionals and laymen.

The professional subculture as the primary social reference on the professional side of the system has been divided in Figure 4 into the basic subsystems of analysis. These divisions indicate the potential areas for research in the sociology of the medical profession. It seems unlikely that the organic subsystem will offer fruitful ground for study, although the male dominance of the profession raises interesting questions related to this sphere. The psychological characteristics of the profession and the comparative psychological profiles of physicians in various medical specialties are beginning to be studied. Within the social subsystem several structures exist, all of which are receiving the attention of sociologists. The medical school,[35] the hospital,[36] the professional societies,[37] structure and types of medical practice,[38] and the relations of physicians to other medical and paramedical groups all fall under this rubric. At the cultural level it is beginning to be recognized that medical professionals, through vocational selection and socialization, represent distinctive patterns of meaning and value. Parsons has spoken of an "optimistic bias" and a "bias in favor of operating" as characterizing the medical profession.[39] Training of future physicians for dealing with uncertainty and for exhibiting "detached concern" has been described by Fox.[40] The ideological superstructure of the profession has been characterized as individualistic, authoritarian (the "doctor's orders" syndrome), and oriented to instrumental activism, but a much more systematic study of professional ideology is needed.

Having discussed the lay actor's individual socio-cultural complex and family as his primary social reference and then the physician's (or physician-surrogate's) individual socio-cultural complex and the medical profession as his primary social reference, we have one task remaining. That is to set the entire system in a total cultural framework. We shall now briefly consider this final factor.

e. *The Total Cultural Framework of the System*. Parsons, in his article on "Definitions of Health and Illness in the Light of American Values and Social Structure" has argued that American medicine must be understood in terms of American value patterns.[41] The Weberian categories of "activism," "worldliness," and "instrumentalism" describe dominant American patterns. These value orientations along with the high level of differentiation have permitted the clear isolation of medicine as a high priority undertaking. Parsons argues:

> ...Both by virtue of its value system, and by virtue of the high level of differentiation of its social structure, American society has been one in which it could be expected that the problem of health, and within this more particularly of mental health, would become particularly salient.[42]

Fox has offered an analysis of American society which illustrates the social and cultural characteristics which promote medical research on human subjects.[43] She demonstrates that economic resources are only one factor. Other factors include the pool of knowledge available, the "strong intellectual, practical, and moral commitment to clinical medical research," and the development of conducive colleague relationships with investigators and subjects. Glazer has recently given an analysis of medical care in Western society in which he argues

that the belief and value system provided by Christianity and
its secularized counterparts have provided a legitimation of
the treatment process to a unique extent.[44] He also finds social structural characteristics upon which the success of the
Western medical tradition is based, factors such as an induc-
tive and empiricist spirit, the body-soul dichotomy, technical
inventiveness, and bureaucratic organization.

The study of the cultural context of a medical action system really leads one to the study of medical anthropology. For
example, deCraemer and Fox found that medical action in the
Congo could not possibly be understood outside of careful consideration of the socio-cultural framework.[45] Medical systems
growing out of the "magical world view," folk culture, non-
Western societies, and the modern West offer radically differing frameworks for a medical action system. We have represented this factor in our unified model in Figure 4 by placing the
entire action system inside a total socio-cultural framework
which is shared by and normally unquestioned by professional
and layman alike.

B. ROLE DESCRIPTIONS IN A UNIFIED THEORY

We have now completed the border of our puzzle. The basic
framework of a unified medical action system has been outlined.
There are, however, several more pieces which we can place.
Specifically, the role descriptions, the analysis of symbol
types which come to us from the sociology of knowledge, and the
pattern variable schema can now be placed within this basic
frame of reference.

Turning first to the role descriptions we encounter the
"sick role," one of the few basic theoretical tools in the sociology of medicine. First proposed by Parsons it is a description of the role expectations for the lay actor.[46] Western, and more specifically American, medicine, to which we
shall limit our discussion, is characterized by a high level of
structural differentiation of types of deviance. Illness is a
partially legitimated form of deviance which has its primary
locus in the organic sphere. It contrasts with deviance in
commitments to collectivities, social forms of deviance from

norms of legality, and cultural forms of deviance from values
and meaning or morality.[47] The diagramming of our analysis of
the lay actor in Figure 4 suggests these possible types of deviance. With increasing differentiation and professionalization of the role of technical specialist we are seeing the
emergence of professional advisors related to each of these potential loci of deviance. The formal institutionalization of
professional specialists is proceeding at different rates for
different forms of specialization. The medical professional is
one of the most highly developed.[48]

Although these distinctions in types of deviance and their
corresponding types of differentiation at first appear to be
nothing more than social scientific description of a modern
highly differentiated society, further reflection reveals that
these theoretical constructions are abstractions, abstractions
which are particularly compatible with certain of the positions
we identified in our introductory survey of the *Werturteilsstreit*. The theoretical constructions support the positions
which are dependent upon the possibility of maintenance of role
separation. The differentiation of types of deviance into
those which are organic from those of other spheres including
those of the moral and religious is a modern sociological example of the dichotomizing effects of the Ionians. Among those
we have labelled the integrators, those who base their integration on the development of particularized professional responsibilities also maintain the necessity of differentiation of
roles. Parsons' suggestion that professional specialists are
related to the differentiation of independent types of deviance
is an example of this role separation. Thus, this theoretical
construction is not without its ideological significance.
There is currently arising a critique of this isolation of
types of deviance from the radical integrationists in the field
of psychiatry. The conceptualization of "mental illness" as a
psycho-organic disease, according to the radical critique, is a
socially acceptable way of disguising and legitimating moral
judgments. Morton Schatzman argues that role separation has
permitted the Western man to take behavior previously thought
to be "bad, criminal, malicious, sinful, selfish, immature,

foolish, [and] idiotic" and redefine it in scientific categories which provide a rationalization for continued disapproval
through the category of psycho-organic deviance which is, as
Parsons points out, a socially legitimated form of deviance.
Schatzman claims:

> The tradition of scientific medicine teaches
> the doctor to keep distinct his moral attitude
> toward diseased persons from his non-moral ob-
> jective attitude towards their diseases. But
> the *moral* views of western society define for
> a psychiatrist what persons he may diagnose as
> "mentally ill" and whom he may treat. A psy-
> chiatrist, especially if he works in a mental
> hospital, is concerned with surveying morals and
> mediating rules. He must deny this if he wishes
> to believe that he adheres to the principles of
> scientific medicine.[49]

Schatzman, Szasz, and others arguing for the radical integration of the scientific and the evaluative would reject any
possibility of isolation of psycho-organic from moral and religious deviance.

The "sick role" is nothing more than a description of the
role expectations of one whose primary locus of deviation is
perceived to be in the organic sphere.[50] There exists an exemption from normal social role responsibilities, an exemption
from responsibility for the condition, an obligation to try to
get well, and an obligation to seek competent help.

Here once again we must pause to distinguish between the
possibility of providing a theoretical formulation describing
a role and the particular efforts at the description which may
have certain ideological biases. In its standard form the sick
role is often presented in a way which is a thinly disguised
defense of the maintenance of the traditional authority and
dominance of the medical professional. Exemption from normal
social role responsibilities is the correlate of the dehumaniz-
ation of the patient into a state of dependency and helplessness. According to Parsons, "By institutional definition of
the sick role the sick person is helpless and therefore in need
of help."[51] One of the most common analogies for the patient-
physician relationship, an analogy we shall criticize in Chapter IV, is that of child to parent. The parental figure is

expected to guide the child in his state of helplessness. "The physician often serves as a court of appeal as well as a direct legitimizing agent."[52]

The second characteristic of the sick role, exemption from responsibility for this condition, exacerbates the condition of helplessness. The patient is viewed as a child exempt from obligations and responsibility. But to take the converse of the slogan that with rights comes responsibilities, many making ideological use of the role description would claim that with loss of obligations and responsibilities comes loss of rights. The patient in fact if not in law loses his rights to make decisions affecting his own life. He is to follow "doctor's orders" even to the extent of submitting himself to custody. He will leave the hospital only when the doctor permits him to. In the extreme case of mental illness legal rights are actually surrendered in the state of utter helplessness so that involuntary institutionalization is made acceptable.

The third characteristic of the sick role, the obligation to try to get well, is the basis of commonly accepted criticism of the "problem patient." By rejecting "doctor's orders" he compounds his organic deviance with social role deviance. The patient who expresses evaluations of appropriate action which are at odds with the medical professional's will be thought of as being in violation of his role expectations. This provides tremendous support for the authority of the professional.

Finally the fourth characteristic, the obligation to seek technically competent help, can often be used as a means of further reinforcing the dependency relationship. The admitted imbalance in technical competency is permitted to dominate the definition of the relationship. According to Robert N. Wilson, one theorist who most passively reiterates the characteristics of the sick role in a way which supports the interests of a dominant, authoritarian professional relationship:

> The patient in many, if not most, health care interactions assumes a passively dependent posture....[53]

This does not mean, however, that efforts to characterize the sick role need be abandoned. What is needed is formulation

of alternative theoretical constructions which, while they will
never be "value-free," will permit clearer visualization of the
implications of the constructions. We cannot make a full reformulation in this survey; nevertheless, we shall illustrate
the potential for reformulation by examining the claim that the
sick role is characterized by lack of competency.

Wilson concludes that "therapeutic relationships, then,
are usually characterized by a pattern of imbalance of power,
interest, and technical expertness."[54] We would suggest that
this arises from description of the sick role in a manner that
places excessive emphasis upon the technical exchange in the
patient-physician relationship. In the terms of our earlier
discussion, it cannot be denied that the instrumental contribution of the technical expert creates a power imbalance, but
this is to overlook the other components of the interaction.
There are instrumental elements originating from the patient
which carry power with them. We have already suggested that
these components should be developed more consciously. Even if
it can be argued that there is an imbalance of instrumental
power on the part of the professional, this still overlooks the
importance of the non-instrumental component. The legitimate
claim to contribute the expressive components of values and
preferences upon which decisions are based rests largely with
the patient. The physician has a duty as well as self-interest
which leads him to act in the best interests of the patient.
If there is an instrumental imbalance in favor of the professional, there may be an equally important if often overlooked
expressive imbalance in favor of the patient. The sick role
could be described as not only one with the obligation to seek
competent help, but also the right to have one's interests,
values, social loyalties, and preferences respected. This
leads us to a discussion of the role characteristics of the
professional actor.

Parsons and Fox have proposed a role analysis of the professional as the counterpart to the "sick role."[55] Like the
sick role it characterizes the behavioral pattern of the professional actor including the instrumental and expressive aspects, but is functionally specific in the sense that the

primary orientation is to the problem of (organic) illness.
The professional actor has role expectations of permissiveness,
support, refusal of reciprocation through adherence to a professional attitude, and introduction of conditional rewards.[56]

As with the sick role, the characterization of the professional role has been called into ideological service. The
characteristics of support and permissiveness support and permit the maintenance of paternalism which we have seen in the
child-parent analogy. Wilson compares the "manipulation of re-
ward" directly to the child-rearing situation.[57] He describes
the "denial of reciprocity" as necessary to the maintenance of
the "independent terrain" on which the doctor stands.[58] In the
same discussion Wilson has the physician undergo an apotheosis
which is heretical not only in its divination of false gods,
but in its carrying of the dichotomy between the divine and the
human to an extreme beyond even that of the most ardent Jensen-
ist:

> Doctor and patient are entrapped in the mysteries
> of life and their intercourse partakes of a reli-
> gious flavor: no patient in extremity of suffer-
> ing and anxiety can regard the physician as of
> life substance with himself; the curative path and
> the curative agent are necessarily endowed with
> transcendent qualities and approached with ardent
> faith rather than cool resolve....The doctor-
> patient relationship is pervaded by mystical-
> religious elements....[There is a] peculiar de-
> pendence of patient on physician, the giving over
> by one individual to another of critical decisions
> affecting not only the course of life but also in
> some instances possibly survival. In order for
> this extraordinary transaction to occur, the pa-
> tient must view his doctor in a manner far removed
> from the prosaic and the mundane.[59]

Here the physician becomes, not merely the priest of the
gods on high, but their very incarnation. In this modern Arian
controversy surrounding the description of the medical professional role, let us hope that the Athanasians get a thorough
hearing.

There is one major issue which remains an open question in
these ideal-typical role descriptions. We can only raise it in
passing. Mechanic, in a discussion of the "Sick Role Revisited," raises doubts about carrying ideal-typical descriptions

to "absurd extremes" and points to the importance of cultural and subcultural factors in defining medical system roles.[60]   We have limited our discussion to American medicine avoiding part of this trouble, but there still remains another problem.   All careful ideal-type theorists are quick to emphasize the difference between the ideal and the real, everyday world.[61]   There is no direct, logical contradiction between the system *ideal* of collectivity-orientation and the fact that a particular physician is egocentric, profit-seeking, and willing to ignore the patient's best interest.   He merely deviates from the ideal which is maintained by the profession and society.   There is a second level, however, at which this phenomenon of deviation from the ideal-type might challenge the ideal itself.   It may be that because of this some such modifications need to be made in the ideal role descriptions of the actors in the medical action system.   We hope to develop this line of analysis further in the future.

C. THE CULTURAL (SYMBOL) SUBSYSTEM IN DECISION-MAKING

Earlier we pointed out that the primary instrumental component in the professional actor's contribution to the medical system consists of medical knowledge from an intellectual discipline formulated and organized into a set of cognitive symbols.   This systematically organized knowledge is thus part of the professional actor's cultural subsystem.   The sociology of decision-making, and more generally the sociology of knowledge, is a rapidly developing field.   For an analysis of the decision-making function of the medical system we have found Parsons' comments on the cultural system to be very helpful.   He argues that the cultural system "is organized about patterns of the meaning of objects and the 'expression' of these meanings through symbols and signs."[62]   He isolates four elements in the cultural system of symbolization: cognitive symbolization, expressive symbolization, patterns of evaluation, and patterns of the grounding of meaning.   Decision-making can be seen as the interaction of these four types of symbolization.   We have represented the cultural subsystems of the professional and lay actors in this way in Figure 4.

The medical knowledge which is available to the professional through his training is to be seen as one portion of the cognitive symbolization or the "patterns of empirical existential ideas." This is seen in the upper left portion of the cultural subsystems of the actors. The implication here is that decision-making is an individual procedure by each one of the actors. This is true if one is careful to emphasize that the information and preliminary processes leading to decision-making include a complex interchange between the actors. The professional finally must decide what prescriptions to write if any; the layman must finally decide whether or not he is to take the prescribed medication. In both cases, however, these decisions should be strongly influenced by the information which comes from the other actors in the system.

The components of the cultural subsystem, as those of the other subsystems, can be analyzed further into subdivisions to the extent that this is found useful for the proposed area of study. Chapter IV of the present volume will be devoted to a thorough delineation of the evaluative system and discussion of its articulation with the other systems.

D. THE PATTERN VARIABLES IN A UNIFIED THEORY

The final element of theory in sociology of medicine which we shall attempt to integrate into our unified model is the pattern variable scheme presented by Parsons in *The Social System*.[63] The five pairs of pattern variables have become a prime tool for describing the professional role of which the medical professional is an example. While each of the pattern alternatives can be questioned at some point, the basic formulation has withstood the critical scrutiny of two decades of sociological analysis. Our plan in this final section is to examine each of these pattern alternatives by relating it to the unified model of medical action which we have developed in this chapter and which is presented in Figure 4. Having this model in front of us we shall attempt to clarify the meaning of the pattern variables and remove some of the ambiguities which have arisen.

1. *Affective Neutrality.*

We shall look at the pattern alternative of affective neutrality first, since it provides a model for the ambiguities of
which we are speaking. The medical professional is continually
placed in intimate contact with individuals in such a way that
emotional involvement could be anticipated. By defining such
situations which might arouse emotional reactions as "professional" a system of sanctions is mobilized which guards against
"inappropriate" reactions.[64] In response to the charge that
affective neutrality makes the physician a cold, insensitive
instrument, Parsons has given credit to Doctors Renée C. Fox
and Miriam Massey Johnson for clarifying the importance of
"empathy" in the physician's role description.[65] Fox had described this in an article on "Training for Detached Concern."
According to Parsons:

> Indeed, in the "art of medicine" there was included
> a component of "empathy" of feeling for the predi-
> caments of the sick which could amount to partial
> identification....There is, in this respect, a
> duality in the role of the physician, namely, that
> whereas the orientation of affective neutrality
> is paramount, at certain stages and under carefully
> controlled conditions, certain types of affectivity
> are not only permitted, but expected.[66]

In terms of our unified model for medical action, the
concept of affective neutrality, or more accurately, detached
concern, can be analyzed as the ideal-typical insistence on the
complete separation between the expressive and cognitive symbolization of the professional actor. In Parsons' terms:

> It is...important that doctors should not let their
> personal dislikes of particular patients be ex-
> pressed in a poorer level of treatment or even
> positive "punishment."[67]

The same is true for the positive emotional attraction for
the patient whether it be sexual or romantic or purely humanitarian. It is recognized that strong emotional attachment
generates a strong tendency for the expressive component to
interfere with the cognitive. This is the basis for the informal prohibition against treatment of members of one's own
family.

2. *Universalism.*

We shall now turn to the pattern alternative of universalism, which, along with functional specificity, Parsons has described as being the most important in the medical context.[68] We shall endeavor to clarify some ambiguities in this pattern, much as has been done with the term "detached concern" for affective neutrality. Particularistic actions take into account factors which are peculiar to the actors involved in a social relationship. They take account of ethnic, religious, political, linguistic, and familial factors (see Fox's discussion of "Medical Scientists in a Chateau" for an example[69]). Particularism is generally related to the complex of non-organic elements which we have diagrammed on the lay actor's (right) half of Figure 4. But it is vitally important to realize that actions are not particularistic *because* they take these factors into account. If this were the case all contributions of sociology of medicine would be particularistic. If Belgian research funds are distributed on this basis and there are no objective rational reasons for such distribution, we recognize the particularism of such actions. However, if a physician who is treating a difficult diabetic case recognizes that the Southern Italian ethnic background of the patient places her in a position where her role as matriarch of an extended family conflicts with the normally prescribed diabetic diet, and because of this he calls the family into consultation about the therapy, we do not accuse this physician of particularism.[70]

The pattern alternative of universalism is not related to the factors in the lay actor's life which are examined by the professional. It rather refers to the way information is handled by the professional. Universalistic patterns are related to the use of generalized, objective criteria in describing situations. In terms of the model we have developed, the medical system is universalistic if the cognitive symbolization of the professional accurately relates to the layman's condition—including his social condition. It is particularistic if the layman's condition is cognitized not directly, but is "filtered" through the value and meaning systems of the professional. Likewise, the professional's situation must be cognitized

by the layman without inputs from *his* cathectic, value, and
meaning systems if it is to be universalistic. Thus the universalistic pattern is one which relates alter to ego's cognitive formulations in an objective, descriptive, *Wertfrei* manner. The universalistic pattern is thus appropriate for the
"descriptive" aspects of the medical process.

3. *Functional Specificity.*

In some ways functional specificity can be viewed as the
inverse of universalism. Universalism excludes no information
from the layman in the medical system; it does limit severely
the elements on the professional side of the system which are
considered relevant. Functional specificity, on the other
hand, places limitations on the aspects of the layman's life
and environment which are relevant. The medical professional
has developed expertise in matters of health and disease (a
portion of his cognitive symbol system). He is not a generalized "wise man" or a sage. He has developed a special competence to advise the layman about the courses of action for
dealing with a particular type of situation which has a primarily organic locus. Other specialists have developed competence
to deal with other areas.

The medical professional may and should move beyond the
organic factors, but the fact remains that he is the proper
specialist to consult only if the organic (excluding the special case of the psychiatrist) element is the primary locus of
attention. If an interaction of organic and other factors is
involved (as is increasingly recognized to be the case in many
situations), a team of professionals with different areas of
competence would most properly deal with the case--a physician
and marriage counselor or a physician and lawyer, for example.

In our discussion of the sociology of decision-making we
claimed that decision-making was the result of the interaction
of several cultural factors, cognitive, expressive, evaluative,
and existential. The formulation of each of these factors can
be viewed as "functions" in the decision-making process. In
this sense, the professional actor, in contrast to the ideal,
pure, descriptive scientist, is not functionally specific. The

medical professional must not only describe objectively the condition of the patient; he must also "prescribe" a course of action, thereapeutic or preventive. He is an applied scientist whose task does not end with the diagnostic task. This means that he must perform all the "functions" of the decision-making process—although he may be influenced by the non-cognitive contributions of the layman.

This places the professional in a difficult position. We have claimed that the professional role is universalistic *in the descriptive task* (which includes having acquaintance with the available scientific, medical knowledge as well as describing the patient's condition). The cognitive formulations of the professional are not "filtered" through his system of value and meaning. We have also claimed that his role is functionally specific in that it focuses upon a particular primary sphere of issues, but that the decision-making task still requires the professional cultural subsystem. This means that the professional *must* introduce a system of value and meaning into his application of medical science in spite of the fact that his area of special competence is a certain type of cognitive knowledge. He must also introduce questions of value and meaning when he chooses what must be described, what standards of description are to be maintained, and to what extent his observations are to be communicated to the lay actor. The pattern alternative of collectivity-orientation becomes important at this point.

4. *Collectivity Orientation.*

Parsons differentiates the role of the professional from that of other occupations, especially the business man, primarily by the fact that the professional is collectivity-oriented.[71]

> The physician's role clearly belongs to what, in our occupational system, is the "minority" group, strongly emphasizing collectivity-orientation. The "ideology" of the profession lays great emphasis on the obligation of the physician to put the "welfare of the patient" above his personal interests, and regards "commercialism" as the most serious and insidious evil with which it has to contend. The line, therefore, is drawn primarily vis-à-vis "business."[72]

We are not here discussing the real-world deviations from the ideal-type. Figures on average annual incomes have raised questions in some people's minds about the collectivity-orientation of the average physician. The fact remains that *ideally* the professional is collectivity-oriented. This is illustrated by the fact that the same questions are not raised so frequently about businessmen with substantial incomes.

Collectivity-orientation implies a mutual obligation on the part of professional and layman to promote values and goals shared by the collectivity. In this case the primary value is the welfare of the patient. Secondary values include the maintenance of the professional and the promotion of the welfare of others through research and protection from exposure to contagion and the like. In terms of our unified model the collectivity-orientation pattern may be understood as the resultant of the interaction of the systems of value and meaning of the actors in the collectivity. To the extent that the professional is able to carry out his portion of the decision-making process using the system of value and meaning which is that resulting from the shared values and goals of the collectivity, he avoids the problem of introducing his own personal values and meaning into the system. These we had pointed to earlier as problematic because the professional has no particular competence in these spheres.

Two problems arise from the use of values and meaning derived from the collectivity. First in some cases it just is not practical. The professional cannot consult the patient about every decision he makes. The layman is not competent to understand the meaning of the choices and even if he were, the task of consulting on every decision would be tedious, endless, and obstructive. The professional must endeavor to consult with the layman at major points in the decision-making process and faithfully project the layman's views in the more routine decisions. Secondly, even if the professional could carry out the consultation process, he could not always in good conscience exclude his own personal, non-professional values and meaning. The professional person-in-role also exists in other roles--as citizen, as moral man, as father, and so forth. What

should a physician do if by the standard value criteria of the
medical profession (such as protection of life) he believes he
should recommend highly effective birth control to a patient
whom he believes would be eager to have such advice, and yet he
is a loyal member of a religious body which has a code of medical ethics which prohibits him from recommending such a procedure or even from recommending a referral? The sources of the
value-criteria for decision-making by professionally competent,
technical experts we see as one of the great problems of applied science including the medical profession. The first step
toward a solution must be the creation of a more general recognition of the problem on the part of professional and layman
alike.

5. *Achievement.*

The achievement pattern alternative is probably the best
understood characteristic of the medical action system. It is
well recognized that at least one of the primary determinants
of the quality of a physician is the extent of his mastery of
scientific knowledge and technical procedures. Perhaps this
element is even emphasized to the exclusion of other important
variables, variables such as mutual compatability, sensitivity,
and availability.

Parsons, in his description of the physician's role, has
linked the universalistic and achievement patterns together,
speaking of the "universalistic-achievement" structuring.[73]
Through the use of the unified model we have developed we shall
attempt to show how this close connection has existed. Achievement refers to the extent to which one has mastered the cognitive material relevant to the defined area of expertise. This
is related to the portion of the professional cultural subsystem we have labeled cognitive symbolization. It will be recalled that this is the same portion of the professional half
of the system which we identified as relevant to the pattern
alternative of universalism. Achievement refers to the incorporation of information and skills into the cognitive area.
Universalism refers to the incorporation of this information
and skills without "contamination" by the value and meaning

system. It is because these two pattern alternatives relate to
the same component in the medical system that they have become
so closely related. This close identification goes beyond the
medical role to all professional and even all occupational
roles at least as long as one is examining ideal-typical Western occupations.

While there is no doubt that achievement is a centrally
important factor in the medical professional role, and one
which, in principle at least, is clearly understood, there are
two complications. First, as mentioned above, emphasis may be
placed on achievement of technical information and skills to
the exclusion of other important factors. Second, there may
exist serious deviations from the ideal which has been described and these deviations may become difficult to detect.
An achieved position under certain conditions may take on as-
criptive characteristics. Achievement of graduation from medical school and completion of an internship program may be interpreted as certification of perpetual competence. The M.D.,
which at first is an achieved degree, may come to function as
legitimating birth-rights of a second birth. Determination of
competence for a physician several years removed from medical
school performing tasks only indirectly related to those
learned in training is a difficult undertaking.[74] In spite of
these difficulties achievement still remains the most cleary
understood of the pattern variables reviewed.

Having now related the five pattern variable alternatives
to our unified model of the medical action system we have completed the task outlined at the beginning of this section. We
have concluded that while certain ambiguities exist, which we
have attempted to clarify in our discussion, the primary pattern alternatives which Parsons has identified remain valid.
They can and should be integrated in their modified form into
our unified theory of the medical action system.

SUMMARY

Our objective in this chapter has been to review the elements which have become available through the years for a theoretical understanding of the sociology of medicine and to

construct a unified theory of a medical action system which
integrates these diverse elements into one complex, but cohe-
sive, theoretical statement. We began our work by examining
L. J. Henderson's description of the patient and physician as a
social system. We subjected this to three modifications based
on developments in the sociology of medicine since the time it
was written.

We first argued that evidence was available that the actors in the social system had to be generalized so that the
"professional actor"--the medical team, the social complexes of
physicians in group practice, partnerships, informal colleague
networks, and in the limiting case the isolated physician--rep-
resented one portion of the system while the lay actor, frequently an individual, but occasionally a group, represented
another portion. Secondly, we insisted that both the expressive and instrumental exchanges must be viewed as two-way processes. Thirdly, we argued for the inclusion of several socio-
cultural factors in the unified theory. These factors included the lay actor's socio-culture which is a complex construction synthesized from the multiplicity of role involvements of
the layman. We called special attention to the family and the
subcultural tradition represented by the family by calling it
the layman's "primary social reference," and giving special attention to it in the model we constructed. In like manner we
included the professional's non-professional socio-culture
which is similarly a unique construction from a multiplicity of
roles. We then identified the professional group as the "primary social reference" of the professional actor. Finally we
provided for the placement of the entire medical system in a
total cultural framework which was shared by professional and
layman.

In the next section of the chapter we related the role descriptions of the patient and professional to the model and
hinted at the possible necessity of changes in the ideal-typical role descriptions on the basis of ideological overtones of
the present constructions and the existence of deviations from
the ideal. Next we brought to bear the work in the sociology
of knowledge by analyzing the cultural subsystem into elements

necessary for the decision-making process: the cognitive, expressive, evaluative and existential.

In the final section we reviewed the pattern variable description of the medical system relating each to our unified model. Affective neutrality depends on the proper separation of expressive and cognitive symbolization and as such is best referred to as detached concern. Universalism describes the relation of the total relevant lay portion of the system, including the socio-cultural elements, to the cognitive symbolization of the professional without "filtering" through his value and meaning system. Functional specificity describes the fact that the professional has competence to deal with problems that have their primary locus in only one portion of the lay side of the system. It does not restrict the elements in the professional's cultural subsystem used in the decision-making process. Collectivity-orientation describes the commitment to the collectivity which produces an interaction of value and meaning systems which the actors use when it is practically possible and when it is consistent with their other role requirements. Finally achievement describes the emphasis placed on the obtaining of technical information and skills by the professional.

It is our hope that in the construction of this unified theory we shall provide a scheme for the recognition and development of areas for further study in the sociology of medicine. In the next chapter we shall take up one component of this unified model, the evaluative subsystem, and explore it in detail.

[1]A note on the methods for resolving conflicts in methodology is in order at this point. Often those who are sophisticated in the study of methodology and the importance of method and theory selection for scientific work will resort to multiple methods much as we have done. There is a danger here, however, one which we shall call the fallacy of consensus of expert opinion when we offer our analysis of the types of value inputs into the scientific process in Chapter IV.

One of the more interesting discussions on the relation of theory to the scientific enterprise and the value components in the selection of theory is in an unpublished paper by G. Burch entitled "The Use of the Proper Theoretical Models in the Scientific Study of Religion" in which she contrasts the stability interaction models of the action system theorists with the conflict models of Hobbes, Marx, C. Wright Mills, and others. After delineating the implications of each for scientific study of religion she then poses the question of selection of a theory for one's work. She proposes that the only solution is to become aware of the merits and shortcomings of each theory and to make use of them in different mixtures depending upon the nature of the problem being studied.

The problem here is that we need a theory for resolving the problem of selecting between the stability-integration model and the conflict-change model. She has said that what we need to do is integrate the theories into a compatible whole. It should be apparent that she has opted totally for one model (the integration model) for the resolution of her meta-dilemma over the selection of theories. It might have been said that the two theories were "inevitably in conflict" and the problem could never be resolved.

In our theoretical formulation we are making the same choice Mrs. Burch did; we are combining theoretical approaches in order to glean the benefits of each. But never let it be said that this is a more scientific approach, or *of necessity* a better attempt to resolve the problem of two conflicting approaches by assuming that the "correct" approach is to be found in a consensus or middle ground position somewhere between the two extremes. It may be that one of the extremes, even the isolated minority, holds the answer; this has been the case in a great many important scientific discoveries. Even more important, the consensus approach is built upon the assumption that the "correct" answer must be drawn from the continuum between the positions under consideration. This excludes all other options. In our present case to attempt a consensus or compromise by making use of both stability-integration and conflict-change models excludes the many other theoretical options which are now available (social interactionist) or could be developed in the future.

[2]L. J. Henderson, "Physician and Patient as a Social System," *New England Journal of Medicine*, CCXII (1935), pp. 819-23.

[3]Samuel W. Bloom, *The Doctor and His Patient* (New York: The Russell Sage Foundation, 1963).

[4]Robert N. Wilson, "Patient-Practitioner Relationships," in *Handbook of Medical Sociology*, ed. by Howard E. Freeman, Sol Levine, and Leo G. Reeder (Englewood Cliffs, N.J.: Prentice-Hall, Inc., 1963), pp. 273-95.

[5]Talcott Parsons, *The Social System* (New York: The Free Press, 1951), pp. 438, 454-65.

[6]*Ibid.*, pp. 436-37.

[7]*Ibid.*, p. 314.

[8]Robert K. Merton, George Reader and Patricia L. Kendall, eds., *The Student Physician* (Cambridge: Harvard University Press, 1957). H. S. Becker, Blanche Greer, E. V. Hughes and A. L. Strauss, *Boys in White* (Chicago: University of Chicago Press, 1961).

[9]Talcott Parsons, "An Approach to the Sociology of Knowledge," in *Sociological Theory and Modern Society* (New York: The Free Press, 1967), pp. 139-65.

[10]L. J. Henderson, "The Practice of Medicine as Applied Sociology," *Transactions of the Association of American Physicians*, LI (1936), pp. 3-22.

[11]L. J. Henderson, "Physician and Patient as a Social System," pp. 820-21.

[12]Samuel W. Bloom, *The Doctor and His Patient*, p. 53.

[13]Eliot Friedson, "The Organization of Medical Practice," in *Handbook of Medical Sociology*, p. 302.

[14]Oswald Hall, "Types of Medical Careers," *American Journal of Sociology*, LV (1949), pp. 243-55.

[15]Edwin P. Jordan, ed., *The Physician and Group Practice* (Chicago: Year Book Publishers, Inc., 1958).

[16]Eliot Friedson, *Patients' Views of Medical Practice* (New York: Russell Sage Foundation, 1961).

[17]Eliot Friedson, "The Organization of Medical Practice," pp. 306-07.

[18]Herman G. Weiskotten, *et al.*, "Trends in Medical Practice--An Analysis of the Distribution and Characteristics of Medical College Graduates, 1915-1950," *Journal of Medical Education*, XXXV (1960), pp. 1071-1121.

[19]Oswald Hall, "The Informal Organization of the Medical Profession," *Canadian Journal of Economics and Political Science*, XII (1946), pp. 30-41.

[20]L. J. Henderson, "Physician and Patient as a Social System," p. 821.

[21]*Ibid.*, p. 820.

[22]*Ibid.*, p. 821.

[23]Robert F. Bales, *Interaction Process Analysis* (Cambridge: Addison-Wesley Press, 1950).

[24]Eliot Friedson, "The Sociology of Medicine: A Trend Report and Bibliography," *Current Sociology*, X-XI, No. 3 (1961-62).

[25]Samuel W. Bloom, *The Doctor and His Patient*, p. 62.

[26]*Ibid.*, p. 256.

[27]Peter Berger and Thomas Luckmann, *The Social Construction of Reality: A Treatise in the Sociology of Knowledge* (Garden City, New York: Doubleday, 1966).

[28]See Bloom, *The Doctor and His Patient*, p. 62. Many studies have indicated the importance of ethnic, or what some have termed subcultural factors, in the definition of the meaning of medical conditions. See Earl Koos, *The Health of Regionville: What the People Thought and Did About It* (New York: Columbia University Press, 1954); Mark Zbrowski, "Cultural Components in Response to Pain," *Journal of Social Issues*, VIII (1952), pp. 16-30; and I. Zola, "Problems of Communication, Diagnosis, and Patient Care," *Journal of Medical Education*, XXXV (1963), pp. 829-38.

[29]Talcott Parsons, *The Social System*, pp. 447-51; Renée C. Fox, *Experiment Perilous* (Glencoe: The Free Press, 1959), pp. 28-29; Renée C. Fox, "Training for Uncertainty," in *The Student Physician*, ed. by Robert K. Merton, George Reader, and Patricia Kendall, pp. 207-43.

[30]Mary Jean Cornish, Florence A. Ruderman, and Sydney S. Spivack, *Doctors and Family Planning* (New York: National Committee on Maternal Health, Inc., 1963).

[31]David Mechanic, *Medical Sociology: A Selective View* (New York: The Free Press, 1968), p. 180.

[32]*Ibid.*, pp. 181-82.

[33]This is not to minimize the important differences which exist in these factors. We are currently seeing increasing innovation and differentiation in medical school curricula.

[34]Temple Burling, Edith Lentz, and Robert N. Wilson, *The Give and Take in Hospitals* (New York: Putnam, 1956); Renée C. Fox, *Experiment Perilous*, pp. 251-53.

[35]Merton, *The Student Physician*; Becker, *Boys in White*; Freat J. Lyden, J. Jack Geiger, and Osler Peterson, *The Training of Good Physicians* (Cambridge: Harvard University Press, 1968).

[36]Harvey L. Smith, "Two Lines of Authority," in *Patients, Physicians and Illness* (Glencoe, Ill.: The Free Press, 1958); Emily Mumford and J. K. Skipper, *Sociology in Hospital Care* (New York: Harper and Row, 1967); Alfred H. Stanton and Morris S. Schwartz, *The Mental Hospital* (New York: Basic Books, 1954).

[37]Oliver Garceau, *The Political Life of the American Medical Association* (Cambridge: Harvard University Press, 1941); Richard Harris, *A Sacred Trust* (New York: New American Library, 1967).

[38]Eliot Friedson, "The Organization of Medical Practice."

[39]Talcott Parsons, *The Social System*, pp. 465-66.

[40]Renée C. Fox, "Training for Uncertainty."

[41]Talcott Parsons, "Definitions of Health and Illness in the Light of American Values and Social Structure," in *Patients, Physicians and Illness*, pp. 165-87, especially, p. 178.

[42]*Ibid.*, p. 181.

[43]Renée C. Fox, "Some Social and Cultural Factors in American Society Conducive to Medical Research on Human Subjects," in *Clinical Investigation in Medicine: Legal, Ethical and Moral Aspects*, ed. by Irving Ladimer and Roger W. Newman (Boston: Boston University Law Medicine Research Institute, 1963).

[44]William A. Glazer, "Medical Care: Social Aspects," in *International Encyclopedia of the Social Sciences*, X, 95-96.

[45]Willy deCraemer and Renée C. Fox, *The Emerging Physician* (Standard, California: The Hoover Institution, 1968).

[46]Parsons, *The Social System*, pp. 436-37.

[47]Parsons, "Definitions of Health and Illness," p. 173.

[48]Talcott Parsons, "Mental Illness and 'Spiritual Malaise'," in *Social Structure and Personality* (New York: The Free Press, 1964), pp. 292-324.

[49]Morton Schatzman, "Morals and Madness," *The Radical Therapist*, I, No. 4 (October-November, 1970), pp. 11-15.

[50]Mental illness represents a special case. Here the deviance is a psychological one rather than organic, although this distinction is extremely difficult to maintain in practice in the era of organic psychoses and organic chemotherapies. The "sick role" must accordingly be modified for this special case, especially with regard to the obligations assigned to the sick person.

[51]Parsons, *The Social System*, p. 439.

[52]*Ibid.*, p. 436.

[53]Robert N. Wilson, *The Sociology of Health: An Introduction* (New York: Random House, 1970), p. 15.

[54]*Ibid.*, p. 16.

[55]Talcott Parsons and Renée C. Fox, "Illness, Therapy, and the Modern Urban American Family," in *Patients, Physicians and Illness*, pp. 234-45, see p. 242; see also Talcott Parsons, *The Social System*, p. 314.

[56]Parsons and Fox, "Illness, Therapy, and the Modern Urban American Family," p. 242. Cf. Parsons' modifications in terminology in "Definitions of Health and Illness in the Light of American Values and Social Structure," p. 566, note 24.

[57]Wilson, *The Sociology of Health*, p. 19.

[58]*Ibid.*, p. 20.

[59]Wilson, *The Sociology of Health*, p. 20.

[60]Mechanic, *Medical Sociology*, pp. 173, 163.

[61]Parsons, *The Social System*, pp. 473-74.

[62]Parsons, "An Approach to the Sociology of Knowledge," p. 141. See also Talcott Parsons, "Pattern Variables Revisited," in *Sociology Theory and Modern Society*, pp. 192-219, especially pp. 205-07.

[63]Parsons, *The Social System*, pp. 434, 438, 454-65.

[64]Parsons, *The Social System*, p. 458.

[65]Talcott Parsons, "Some Theoretical Considerations Bearing on the Field of Medical Sociology," in *Social Structure and Personality* (New York: The Free Press, 1967), pp. 325-58, especially p. 336.

[66]Parsons, "Medical Sociology," p. 336.

[67]Parsons, *The Social System*, p. 459.

[68]Parsons, "Medical Sociology," p. 329.

[69]Renée C. Fox, "Medical Scientists in a Chateau," *Science*, CXXXVI (1962), pp. 476-83.

[70]See Bloom, *The Doctor and His Patient*, pp. 37-50 for a discussion of a case.

[71]It should be noted that since *The Social System*, Parsons, in "Pattern Variables Revisited," pp. 192-219, has argued

that collectivity-orientation is not a pattern variable in the same sense as the other four pairs, but is a duality of a different type. We have nevertheless included it in our discussion here because of its importance in understanding the professional role.

[72]Parsons, *The Social System*, p. 435.

[73]Parsons, *The Social System*, p. 454.

[74]See Lois Hoffman, "How do Good Doctors Get That Way?" in *Patients, Physicians and Illness*, pp. 365-81. See also Freat J. Lyden, *et al.*, *The Training of Good Physicians*.

CHAPTER III

THE SPHERE OF EVALUATION

We now have before us a model of the action system in
which scientific and technological decisions are made. We took
the liberty of simplifying the discussion by referring to the
medical action system as an example of the interaction between
the professional with competence in a specific area of scientific and technological knowledge and the lay actor. The model
is, however, applicable to any professional-lay action system.
Certain pieces would have to be modified: the specific role descriptions would change, the characteristics of the professional actor's primary social reference would be somewhat different
for other scientific disciplines but the system--the factors
that one would have to consider to perform a complete analysis
of the decision-making process--are essentially the same.

It is the purpose of this chapter to narrow our focus to
the structure of the sphere of evaluation of the cultural subsystem of the actors. There are three themes that will be developed in the chapter. First we shall continue in the style
of Chapter II to analyze the components of the action system by
characterizing the categories of the sphere of evaluation on
the basis of the reference for evaluation. Second, using the
categories we have described, we shall differentiate levels of
generality in the process of evaluation, coining the concept of
"Cultural Value Complex" as the resultant evaluation for a
given specific issue area. Third, we shall argue that certain
elements of evaluation, those which are of ultimate significance, are essentially religious.

A. CATEGORIES OF EVALUATION

Although the concept of value is ancient, the systematic
study of value and evaluation and the formation of a generalized theory of evaluation is a quite recent phenomenon. It is
not the purpose of this chapter to develop a general theory of
value or even present a review of such theories. These are
available in the literature.[1] In the first part of this

91

chapter we shall present a particular type of classification of
values which will be helpful in our analysis of the value factors in scientific and technological decision-making. Nicholas
Rescher, in his *Introduction to Value Theory*, has summarized
six main principles for classification values: subscribership,
the objects at issue, the sort of benefits at issue, the sort
of purposes at issue, the relationships between subscriber and
beneficiary, and the relationship of value to other values.[2]
Other bases for classification are described in the literature.[3]

The first principle of classification described by
Rescher, subscribership, distributes values on the basis of the
response to the question, "Is the value held--or is it such
that it ought to be held--by a person or by a group, and then
what sort of group?" The classification we shall present resembles Rescher's subscribership classification in that it differentiates among personal, group, (and in our case universal)
values, but unlike Rescher we shall focus not on the subscriber, but on the reference for the legitimation of the evaluation.

Culture is that part of life which is distinguished by the
property of being intrinsically transmissible from one social
unit, from one personality or social system to another. It is
comprised of symbols which are meaningfully integrated into an
ideational system. Symbol systems of culture, as we have indicated in Chapter II, can be cognitive, expressive, meaning
grounding, and evaluative.

The evaluative system is made up of units or values which
Clyde Kluckhohn defines as "conceptions, explicit or implicit,
distinctive of an individual or characteristic of a group, of
the desirable which influence the selection from available
modes, means, and ends of action."[4] Let us being with Wolfgang
Köhler's characterization of the phenomenological theory of
value.

We are handicapped somewhat by Köhler's shifting terminology. He begins by defining value as "the trait of intrinsic
requiredness or wrongness."[5] This is an acceptable, if somewhat restrictive, definition. A problem arises, however, when,
under the influence of Ralph Barton Perry, he also equates

value to interest which in turn is related to conation, tendency, and striving.[6]

What is at stake is the character of the "vector" or directional force which Köhler and other Gestalt psychologists identify with the experience of value. Specifically, there is a question of the intensity of this vector force. Köhler, by subsuming all vector forces of the phenomenal field under the category of requiredness minimizes the variations in the intensity of the vector. Mandelbaum, on the other hand, is more precise. He differentiates from among all those phenomena characterized by conation certain ones which place a *demand* on us.[7] Some actions are willed, and explicitly considered valuable according to Mandelbaum, when they are nothing more than preferences. Such actions as cutting my hair today, going to the movies tomorrow, or rereading a novel he cites as examples. Other phenomena are characterized by a demand quality so that we are obliged, or bound, to act.[8] This differentiates preferences from obligations. It would seem more appropriate and in accord with common usage to distinguish between requiredness and the more general vectoral phenomenon of value.

We have noted that, for Köhler, the first characteristic of value is that it is experienced as a vector.[9] Value aspects of the phenomenal field have "direction or directedness." Then, beyond that according to Köhler, "interest as a vector is experienced as issuing from a definite part of the field."[10] Finally, "interest or striving is directed toward the phenomenal object in question."[11]

One of the great strengths of Köhler's phenomenological description is that it avoids completely, at this point in his analysis, the claim that the vector originates from the self. In his terms the subjectivistic theory of values "would appear to be at least incomplete." In a slip into scientific heresy he shows his concern for the layman's quest to move beyond the subjectivistic theory. He says:

> Personally I understand this objectivistic attitude
> of the layman very well because I find myself exactly in his position.[12]

Köhler, in his description of values as phenomena, states that they are experienced as originating as vectors in parts of contexts and extend toward others with a quality of acceptance or rejection.[13] He stresses over and over again that the part of the context from which the vector originates is not always the self. He claims:

> In this formulation I have not explicitly mentioned the self as being the source of the vector....So far we have found two classes of contexts, in which there is requiredness. In the first the vector points toward the object, in the other the object is the point of origin of the vector....That in many examples such vectors issue from the self is a relatively minor point. Its discussion does not belong in the interpretation of requiredness as such.[14]

This distinction in the sources of the vector force will be the basis of our classification of values for the present discussion. In more sociological terms these vector forces can be viewed as the bases for legitimation of the evaluative claim.

Among systems of evaluation there are many bases for legitimation of the values, many sources to which appeal can be made to support the evaluation. The general form of an evaluative statement is "X is evaluated positively (negatively)" or "X is good (bad)" or "You ought (not) to do X." When defense of the evaluative statement is demanded, a first response typically is the citation of the reference of the legitimation.

As we present the classification it will become apparent that the reference for legitimation is extremely significant for the decision-making process. Only when there is some understanding and agreement on the reference for legitimation can there be any basis for selecting the appropriate decision-makers. Needless to say, the bases for legitimation are not mutually exclusive. Some evaluations may normally be legitimated at one level, but when challenged the evaluator may shift his claims to a higher level of generality. Further, in any given decision-making situation, there will be evaluations required which appeal to more than one of the bases of legitimation. In Parsonian language there exists a hierarchy of control which is crucial for ranking the claims to legitimation.[15] Normally and other things being equal, the higher in the hierarchy of control a claim for legitimation, the more precedence

it is given. Appeal to personal desire, even when extremely
intense, is normally subordinated to a directly conflicting appeal to law or truth or morality. We shall present our categories of evaluation in order of ascending hierarchy of control. The classification is presented schematically in Figure
5.

1. *Personal Legitimation.*

At the lowest level of control X might be "good" simply
because the speaker (evaluator) approves of X or because X is
believed to lead to some satisfaction which the speaker hypo-
thetically desires. In the medical context, cosmetic surgery
is easily recognized as having primarily personal legitimation.
Many other choices, however, when analyzed carefully, are seen
to be rooted primarily at this level, e.g., the use of birth
control ("every child a wanted child") and the selection of
birth control methods from those thought to be moral and "sufficiently" safe and effective. Kant terms imperatives which
declare a possible action to be practically necessary as a
means of attaining something else that one may will "hypothetical."[16] Hypothetical imperatives tend to be viewed as personally legitimated and many of them are, but this is not the distinguishing characteristic of personal legitimation. The
unique feature is that the value is a conception of the desirable which is not grounded beyond the self. In the phenomenol-
ogist's terms, the vector has its origins in the self. The intensity of the vector is also not the necessary distinguishing
feature. Preference (in contrast to obligations in Mandelbaum's terminology) tend to be viewed as originating in the
self, but the demand quality which is characteristic of obligation is not necessarily suprapersonal.

There is a metaethical correlate of this personal basis of
legitimation. The personal relativism of someone like Edward
Westermarck is based on the view that rightness *means* nothing
more than that X arouses or tends to arouse an emotion of approval in the speaker.[17] It is important to realize, however,
that rightness as an *ethical* concept means something quite different from this and still maintain that *some* values are

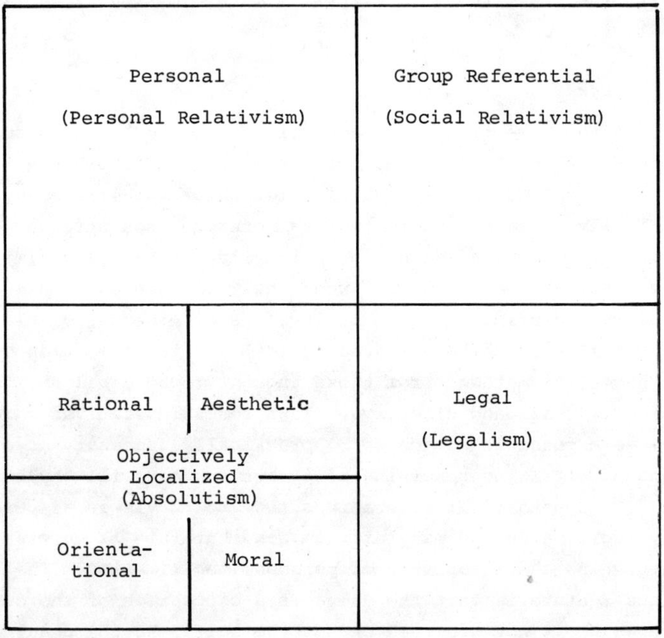

Fig. 5. The Categories of Evaluation

legitimated at no higher level of generality than the self.
Personal relativism grew out of a period when many evaluations
which were formerly taken to be suprapersonally legitimated
(e.g., opposition to alcoholic consumption, card playing, or
sexual deviance) were being shifted down in the hierarchy of
control to lower levels of legitimation. This need not mean,
however, that *all* evaluations are legitimated at this level.

If one is involved in a decision-making situation, one
element of the evaluation will be personally legitimated values.
It is incumbent upon the professional and lay actors to permit
a maximization of these values--in so far as they do not conflict with others higher in the hierarchy of control.

2. *Group Referential Legitimation.*

A second reference for legitimation depends on a cathexis
for a group to which the speaker can refer for legitimation.
The assumption of a group referential legitimation is a common
group loyalty. The loyalty to the group is deemed to be sufficient legitimation of the customs, folkways or mores of the
group. In spite of the fact that the reference extends beyond
the speaker, it is clearly recognized that the level of trans-
cendence of the evaluative reference is low. If the statement
"You *ought* not dress your baby boy in pink (or ought to bind
your feet or raise a small family) because members of our society, social class, etc. do this" is questioned, both the
speaker and the questioner tend to recognize that there is no
legitimation beyond reference to the group or to personal ad-
vantages that might accure by conforming to the group's standards.

We are now discovering inconsistencies in group customs
which give rise to questions about the religious and moral rationalization of social patterns. In a recently completed
study, Puerto Ricans in New York City were found to have a social pattern of female sterilization as a means of birth control once the desired number of children had been born. While
this was practiced routinely in Puerto Rico, in New York City
it met strong resistance by Anglo-Saxon, middle-class physicians practicing in local hospitals. They would condone

sterilization only in extreme circumstances--generally on radical medical grounds or when the product of a woman's age and her number of live offspring equalled 120.[18]

The implication of this observation is that the primary distinction in the evaluations is one of group identification. The repeated discovery that group loyalty is related to evaluations particularly during expansionist periods of history (such as the Greek and Western expansion) has given rise to a corresponding metaethical theory. Theorists such as William Graham Sumner hold a position that the statement "X is right" *means* nothing more than that "X is approved by the speaker's society or social group."[19] It should be clear, however, that the observation that *some* behavior is legitimated by a cathexis for a social group or even that outside observers can correlate certain evaluations with group identification, does not mean that *all* evaluations are reduced to group referential legitimation.[20]

3. *Legal Legitimation.*

A marginal case with somewhat greater phenomenological objectivity is the reference to a positive legal system as a source of legitimation. A society's legal system functions as a basic source of integration. There is a clear perception of a distinction between the group's customs and the legal system. The claim "X is wrong because it is illegal" carries substantially more weight than the claim that it is a violation of a custom. The basis for this is complex. Phenomenologically, appeal to illegality is perceived as more "objective" than a simple group referential appeal. This is possibly linked to an implied "moral" evaluation, i.e., that it is morally wrong to violate the legal code of a society in which one has, by previous actions, implied faithfulness to that society. (Socrates was not unaware of the principle.)

Nevertheless rejection of an appeal to (positive) legality is still recognized either in the name of a higher moral principle or by simple rejection of the authority of the society in question. Thus appeal to legality is not categorical.

We noted that when personally legitimated values were at stake in a decision-making process, the appropriate action was to "consult the expert," i.e., the persons whose values were most directly involved. For values of legal legitimation, likewise, one would appropriately consult the expert on questions of the law (in so far as the legal issues are not well known to the decision-makers).

4. *Objectively Localized Legitimation.*

Finally there is a type of evaluation which is phenomenologically quite different from the types we have already described. The first category was characterized by a vector which originated from the self. The second and third categories have vector forces which are suprapersonal in their origin, but still arise from a particular social point in the phenomenological context, the social group. With objectively localized legitimation we reach the highest level of generalization, the highest level in the hierarchy of control. In response to the question why a logically valid syllogism is to be valued there is not a direct response. It is "just in the nature of things." The legitimation of the value of truth transcends any particular portion of the phenomenological context. The demand quality is perceived as a fitting part of the *whole* suprapersonal objective order as it exists independently of not only the self but also other persons or groups.[21] The vector is perceived as being "objective" in its origin in the sense of coming from the whole of the suprapersonal order, transcending any personal or social sources.

As Dyck has pointed out, characterizing the vector as an objective, impersonal demand quality is not sufficient to delineate it as a moral demand.[22] This describes a larger group of evaluations which claim objectively localized legitimation. These we have diagrammed in the lower left-hand quadrant of Figure 5.

Within the evaluative subsystem we have thus far differentiated categories of evaluation in ascending order of the hierarchy of control from the personal which has a primarily adaptive function to the objectively localized which, as the highest order of legitimation functions to maintain the basic grounding of value. Thus within the evaluative subsystem there

is a strict parallelism to the functional differentiation of
the cultural system itself. Now at the level of objectively
localized legitimation we find a third level of functional parallelism. There are, first, objectively localized patterns of
cognitive symbolization which are *valued*; these we call truth.
There are, second, objectively localized patterns of cathexis
which are *valued*; these we call aesthetics. While both of
these are ultimate values which, according to at least many
systems of ethics, one has a moral duty to maximize, still
neither is itself moral.

For an objectively localized, impersonal, demand quality
to be categorized as moral, there must be other conditions.
Dyck has argued convincingly that these characteristics are the
elements of choice and reflexive quality. For the demand to be
considered moral it must present the self with at least two
genuine options for choice.[23] Further the demand must be reflexive; it must be a demand for a response in some fashion or
other.[24] Thus according to Dyck:

> moral requiredness occurs in our phenomenal world
> as an impersonal, objective, and gap induced de-
> mand for some sort of fitting response from the
> self in situations where the self sees itself con-
> fronted by at least two genuine options.[25]

We have thus far accounted for the classical values of
truth, beauty, and goodness. There are both theoretical and
empirical reasons to believe that there remains a final category of evaluation which has been overlooked. From our theoretical construction it is apparent that this final category
should be the value of objectively localized patterns of the
groundings of meaning. A world history of man's religious nature reflected in contemporary literature in volumes such as
Rudolf Otto's *Idea of the Holy* suggests empirically that there
does exist a set of patterns expressing the basic nature of
reality which play a critically important role in any system of
evaluation. This fourth set of "objectively localized" values
should express man's orientation to the maintenance of the most
fundamental grounding of reality. It should include the evaluational component of man's theological, philosophical *Weltanschauung* dealing with such basic patterns as man's relation to

nature and supernature, the goodness of man, and the orientation to past, present and future.

Quite obviously what we are looking for here as the highest level of objectively localized evaluation is what Clyde
Kluckhohn and later Florence Kluckhohn and F. L. Strodbeck have
called "value orientations."[26] According to Clyde Kluckhohn,
value-orientation is a term used for:

> those value notions which are (a) general, (b)
> organized, and (c) include definitely existential
> judgments. A value-orientation is a set of
> linked propositions embracing both value and
> existential elements.[27]

The classification of value orientations by Kluckhohn and
Strodbeck is diagrammed in Figure 6. In doing so we follow the
standard functional scheme which has been used throughout the
last two chapters. The time orientation represents a dimension
not presentable in two-dimensional space. In fact we have already discussed that the functional analysis is most appropriate for a "cross-sectional" or fixed point in time analysis.
This is the basis for the accusation that Parsonian analysis
has a "static bias." In fact all of our theoretical models imply a time dimension. It can be visualized as a linear series
of diagrams which, taken in series, represent the changes in
the system which take place through time. Nevertheless, the
traditional theoretical tools of functional analysis do not
lend themselves to description of change and time functions.
For this reason we have represented the value-orientation related to time in Figure 6 in three dimensional space. In Chapter IV when we want to focus on the dynamic element of the process of scientific and technological decision-making we shall
adopt cybernetic theory for the purpose.

This completes our classification of the categories of
evaluation. In our empirical work we shall attempt to measure
some of these categories which appear to have the most relevance to the specific question we are investigating.

B. THE CULTURAL VALUE COMPLEX

Having analyzed the categories of evaluation, we have
provided greater detail for our unified model for scientific

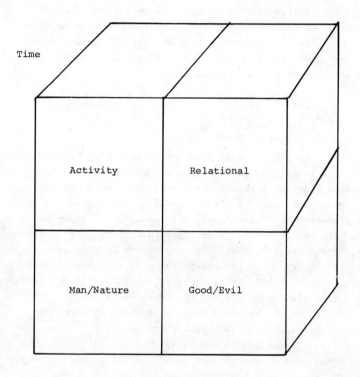

Fig. 6. Orientational Values

and technological decision-making. We still have not, however, approached the crucial question for decision-making analysis: how are the values which have been delineated in the sphere of evaluation brought to bear on a specific decision which has to be made? How do values (rational, aesthetic, moral and orientational) gain specificity such that they can become a component in the decision-making process? This is perhaps one of the most crucial and underemphasized questions in the discipline of ethics. It is the point at which ethicists are most frequently and justifiably attacked.

We have found that it is necessary to make a theoretical differentiation according to the degree of specificity within each of the evaluative categories as well as on the basis of the reference for legitimation. Our point is best illustrated by consideration of the types of questions which arise in the discipline of ethics. The first question of the formal discipline of ethics is meatethics--the question of the meaning of ethical terms and the justification of ethical claims. It is a point beyond which ethicists often never move. The second question is that of normative ethics--the question of what kin kinds of acts are morally right and wrong and what things are ultimately values.

Both of these questions must be dealt with at a high level of generality. Questions of what is ethically required in a specific set of circumstances move us beyond these two areas to questions of casuistry. It is not easy to move from the description of a set of ultimate goods and right-making characteristics to specific ethical judgments about what is a right action in a specific yet complex situation. Because of this the enterprise of casuistry has a tarnished reputation. Most ethicists have abandoned it altogether, yet it is the end point of ethical decision-making. This is one of the reasons why scientists have shied away from formal ethical analysis when they need to make decisions involving ethical considerations. They turn instead to their own methodology--one which is adapted to the specificities of the decision-making situation-- the case study method.

Part of the reason why casuistry has been unsuccessful in the past when it has been attempted by ethicists and moral

theologians is that the gap between affirmation of an ultimate
value or right-making characteristic and a specific moral judgment is a very large one. It is one thing to defend the moral
value, freedom--quite another to argue that every woman must
have the freedom to have an abortion under circumstances x, y,
and z. In an effort to elucidate the leap from generalized
norms to specific moral judgments about specific cases (such as
abortion or oral contraception) we think it is helpful to differentiate two levels of evaluative propositions.

The typical judgments or rules of casuistry are final summary statements, summary rules to use Ramsey's terminology.[28]
To anticipate the illustration we shall use in the second half
of this study, an example of such a final summary statement
would be "The use of oral contraceptives is morally wrong
(right)." Now it is clear that it is a huge step from statements of right-making characteristics such as justice and
reparation and fidelity to this summary rule.

It is possible to establish a secondary set of ethical
judgments which are still content specific, but which provide
more ethical information than the simple summary rule. These
can be determined by analysis of the statements and argumenta-
tion of an ethically relevant subject (such as oral contraception). The final specification of a set of ethical judgments
which collectively feed into the final summary statement can,
under the best conditions, be made more precise by a factor
analysis of empirical measures of ethical judgments, but tentative groupings can be made through content analysis. Once the
secondary set of ethical judgments is determined, the ethicist
has the "missing link" in the transition from generalized norms
to final judgments. With a set of secondary propositions which
have been developed empirically, the task of normative analysis
is simplified. Each item in the set of secondary judgments can
be evaluated in terms of the ultimate goods and right-making
characteristics available from normative ethics. By establishing empirically an intermediate step between the generalized
norms and the gross summary rule the gap has been narrowed and
the specific decision-making process is brought into articulation with the contributions of the discipline of ethics.

Thus far we have described a secondary level of ethical judgments which stands between the norm deficient summary rule and content deficient right-making characteristics and ultimate goods. Likewise, it is possible to formulate a theoretical conception at this secondary level of specificity for all categories of the evaluative process. Taken together these can be thought of as forming what we shall call the "cultural value complex." By Cultural Value Complex we shall mean the resultant of an integrated application of a set of evaluative standards to a specific issue area. The set of ethical judgments at this secondary level of specificity which feed into the final judgment could then be seen as the "ethical factor" or "ethical component" of the Cultural Value Complex. Likewise, there will be rational, aesthetic, and orientational components in the Cultural Value Complex. Thus the complex contains components from all of the value-types we have described.

Why have we chosen to call the value complex "cultural?" Cultural is an ambiguous term which fits the concept we are attempting to construct perfectly. In the first place the term "cultural" might even be seen as redundant in that values as symbolic constructions are of necessity cultural. Evaluative symbolization is a portion of the cultural system of our unified model of the action system. At this point we are merely following well established categories and construction.[29] But secondly, "cultural" implies limited to particular social groups, societies, or cultures. This, of course, is exactly the case whenever one initiates a construction by empirical description of a set of value components on the basis of content analysis of literature and factor analysis of collected data on evaluative judgments.

"Cultural," however, has still a third connotation, one which suggests the link between the description of existing values from which we begin and the evaluation of those values from the perspective of the normative disciplines of ethics, logic, aesthetics, theology, and philosophy. The cultural system, as the term is used by Parsons, is the system highest in the hierarchy of control. Beyond it is the transcendent. It stands in an immediate dialectical relation to ultimate

reality, which Parsons calls the "environment of action" contiguous with the cultural system. The symbolization of the
cultural system which we have termed objectively localized is
grasping beyond itself reaching for the reality which it attempts to reduce to a system of symbols we call language. The
sociologists of religion, Thomas Luckmann and Peter Berger, develop this dimension of Parsons when they talk about the social
(cultural) construction of reality. Man constructs a system of
symbols which constitutes his *Weltanschauung* not willy-nilly,
but because they represent his best effort to form a symbolic
construction of what phenomenologically *is* ultimate reality.
In Berger's terms:

> ...the anthropological ground of these projections
> may itself be the reflection of a reality that *in-
> cludes* both world and man, so that man's ejacula-
> tions of meaning into the universe ultimately point
> to an all-embracing meaning in which he himself is
> grounded....Put simply, this would imply that man
> projects ultimate meanings into reality because
> that reality is, indeed, ultimately meaningful,
> and because his own being (the empirical ground
> of these projections) contains and intends these
> same ultimate meanings.[30]

The symbolic universe of the cultural system, or at least
the objectively localized portions of it, point beyond themselves to an objective, impersonal reality which is the stuff
of normative critique. To say that our Cultural Value Complex
is "cultural" hopefully will continue to convey this critical
normative dimension.

C. THE RELIGIOUS DIMENSION IN THE SYSTEM OF EVALUATION

In the Introduction I suggested that the forces of dualism
and dichotomization were pitted against those of integration,
whether professional or more universal. This dialectic can
also be seen in the discussion of the relation of the religious
to the evaluative. The "value-free" scientist would claim to
avoid incorporation of any "religious" dimension in his decision-making involving scientific and technological issues.
Even the decision-maker who is well aware that he is making decisions involving an ethical dimension will often maintain that
his ethical reasoning is "non-religious."

Those whose orientation is toward isolating values from religion build their case on two dichotomies. We shall examine these in turn.

1. *The Sacred and the Profane.*

After rejecting the characteristics of the supernatural and the idea of God or a spiritual being as definitive for religious phenomena, Emile Durkheim defines religion as:

> a unified system of beliefs and practices relative to sacred things, that is to say, things set apart and forbidden--beliefs and practices which unite into one single moral community called the Church, all those who adhere to them.[31]

For Durkheim the separation is absolute. The sacred and the profane are utterly different.

> In all the history of human thought there exists no other example of two categories of things so profoundly differentiated or so radically opposed to one another.[32]

If the religious is so radically separated from the profane, then it is difficult to maintain that a system of evaluation need have any relation whatsoever to the religious. Of course there may be ethical claims which are religious; there may even be some entire evaluation systems which are rooted in the sacred, but evaluative systems do not necessarily contain a religious dimension.

The radical separation of the sacred and the profane is not, however, the only way of conceptualizing the relation of the religious to the rest of nature.

Thomas Luckmann, building on the theoretical work of Durkheim, differs from him in several significant ways. First, Luckmann separates the notion of the religious from that of the Church, even in the highly generalized sense that Durkheim meant. More important for our purposes, Luckmann rejects the radical dichotomy of the sacred and the profane, preferring instead to view reality and the culturally constructed symbolic universes which are systematic accounts of that reality as more of a continuum. Symbolic universes are, according to Luckmann:

socially objectivated systems of meaning that refer,
on the one hand, to the world of everyday life and
point, on the other hand, to a world that is experienced as transcending everyday life.[33]

Such a symbolic universe which provides an integrated configuration of meaning or a world view as an "objective and historical social reality" performs, according to Luckmann, an essentially religious function. Such a world view is an "elementary social form of religion," a form which, in contrast to the
institutional form of the Church, is universal in human society.[34]

Now the notion of a phenomenologically objective symbol
system which is experienced as transcending everyday life
sounds remarkably akin to the portion of evaluative symbolization which we, following the phenomenologists, termed "objectively localized." While it would be stretching the concept of
a *Weltanschauung* to include the personally, socially, and le-
gally legitimated categories of evaluation, the values which
are legitimated by reference to phenomenologically objective
reality would seem to be not only appropriate to, but an essential part of, the concept. While some rational, aesthetic,
ethical, or orientational values may arise from a specifically
institutional religious context, they all, by their very nature, have an objectivity about them which gives them a religious dimension in this very broad sense of the term. In this
manner the radical separation of the sacred and the profane
collapses.

We can go further than this, however. While, for Luckmann, a *Weltanschauung* has a religious character in this first,
most general and universal sense, it takes on a specific historical social form when the configuration of religious repre-
sentations form a *sacred* universe.[35] This distinction between
a general *Weltanschauung* as a religious phenomenon and a sacred
universe as a specific form need not force one to revert to a
Durkheimian dualism. As a subspecies of the more general form
it cannot.

Tillich's understanding of religion as ultimate concern is
helpful in clarifying both this and the second dichotomy between religion and evaluation which we shall discuss below.
According to Tillich:

> In accordance with their essential nature, moral-
> ity, culture, and religion interpenetrate one
> another. They constitute the unity of the spirit,
> wherein the elements are distinguishable but not
> separable.[36]

Religion, the self-transcendence of life, stands, according to Tillich, in an ambiguous relationship to the sacred and
theprofane, and that ambiguity is contained in Tillich's use of
the term "ultimate."[37] Religion incorporates the quality of
ultimate concern.[38] God is the "name for that which concerns
us ultimately."[39] Ultimate is an important term, one with a
connotation differing greatly from that of the dualistic language of Durkheim. Ultimate, according to the dictionary,
means farthest, most remote, last in a train of progression.
The image is one of a continuum, with an endpoint beyond which
one can go no further. The religious, for Tillich, is not
radically different from the worldly, but a unique extreme of
it. The Tillichian *Weltanschauung* is a unity, distinguishable
but not separable.

This is the same conception we find in Luckmann. We have
noted that for Luckmann the *Weltanschauung* as an objectivated
symbolic universe was a universal form of religion. He, like
Tillich, sets off a portion of the continuum of the symbolic
universe. According to him:

> The world view in its totality was defined earlier
> as a universal and nonspecific social form of
> religion. Consequently, the configuration of
> religious representations that form a *sacred uni-
> verse* is to be defined as a *specific historical
> form of religion.*[40]

Luckmann makes clear that by sacred he means exactly what
Tillich does. It is the sphere of "ultimate significance" distinguished from the trivial by "many graduated strata of meaning."[41] If, as we have argued, the categories of value which
are objectively legitimated are part of religion in its universal form (as part of a *Weltanschauung*), then those portions
of the objectively legitimated system of evaluation--the rational, aesthetic, the ethical, and the orientational--which
are distinguished by their ultimacy can rightly be said to constitute a portion of the sacred (ultimate) universe which is a

specific historical form of religion. As such the system of
evaluation of necessity contains within it the religious dimension. In these terms the notion of a "non-religious" system of
evaluation is possible only when it excludes those values which
are objectively localized, or more narrowly, when it excludes
those values which are ultimate within the categories of value
which are objectively localized.

2. *The Ontological and the Evaluative.*

There is a second dichotomy upon which a separation of the
evaluative and the religious is based. Durkheim, who characterized religion as a unified system of beliefs and practices
relative to sacred things, never suggests that the beliefs and
practices may include those with the vectorial or demand quality which we have said characterizes the evaluative. Talcott
Parsons, student of Durkheim, heightens the dichotomy between
the religious and the evaluative in his theoretical work. For
Parsons religion is that portion within the cultural system
which pertains primarily to symbolization of the grounding of
existential meaning (see Figure 4 in Chapter III).[42] Clyde
Kluckhohn, associate of Parsons in the formulation of the general theory of action, makes the same distinction in his discussion of "normative and existential propositions."[43] He
claims:

> Existence and value are intimately related, inde-
> pendent and yet--at least in the analytical
> level--conceptually distinct.[44]

Yet in Kluckhohn's own words there is strong evidence of
the integrationist themes which he speaks of when he points out
that existence and value are intimately related. The concept
of value-orientation (or orientational value in our terminology
as developed in the last chapter, see Figures 5 and 6) which
Kluckhohn develops reveals this. Value-orientation is the term
used for those values which, among other things, include defi-
nitely existential judgments. A "value-orientation is a set of
linked propositions embracing both value and existential elements."[45]

More generally it can be claimed that there is an existential component in all the categories of evaluation which are objectively legitimated. The notion that evaluation is independent of existence is built on the positivist understanding of value which, as we have seen, has its origins in the dualistic separation of extended substance and mental substance in Descartes, Locke, and the early modern philosophers of science who thought they could separate the "natural" and the "moral." In the next chapter we shall explore this argument more fully. For now we should observe that their position is at least open to question. It cannot be denied, however, that the categories of value which are objectively legitimated form a part, and a very central part, of the *Weltanschauung* which Luckmann has described as an elementary social form of religion. Luckmann himself makes the claim.[46]

The same point is made in Tillich's theological statement of the interpenetration of morality with culture and religion in the statement we quoted above. If Tillich's concept of the ultimate permits us to bridge the dichotomy of the sacred and profane, then his use of the term "concern" in characterizing the quality of the religious, leads him to overcome the dichotomy between the existential and the evaluative. God, the ground of Being, is also that which *concerns* us ultimately. The term concern introduces the vectorial element which we have identified with the evaluative. Morality is the only objectively legitimated category of value with which Tillich deals directly in this context. It shall have to serve as a model of how he relates religion to all of objectively legitimated values. Morality, he says, is essentially related to religion.

> Religion gives to morality the unconditional character of the moral imperative, the ultimate moral aim....[1]

Without the religious element of self-transcendence the objective demand could not be felt. The ultimate moral demand is replaced by conditional hopes and fears which have their origins in psychological and social realms of personal and group legitimations.[48] Tillich along with Luckmann leads us to the conclusion that the system of evaluation contains within it

elements which are essentially religious, elements which are
phenomenologically rooted in the *Weltanschauung* which Luckmann
calls the (universal) elementary social form of religion. More
specifically it contains elements in which the values are ultimate in exactly the sense which Tillich and Luckmann use the
term. The basic distinction between values and the religious
on the basis of the dichotomy of the existential and the evaluative cannot be supported. This is not to say that all the
categories of evaluation are religious in either of these
senses. Those which are only personally or socially legitimated are not. Nor is this to say that some objectively legitimated values cannot be distinguished from others by their
having their roots in institutional religion of the ecclesias-
tic type. Religion as a special, ecclesiastical, social institution is a specific social form of religion. Certainly some
aesthetic, moral, and orientational values have their origin
here while others do not, but this does not in any way minimize
our conclusion that *every* system of evaluation which includes
objectively legitimated components contains a religious dimension in the broader sense in which Tillich and Luckmann use the
term.

This completes our analysis of the system of evaluation.
Placing this element of the analysis in its place in the unified theory of the scientific and technological action system
system we constructed in Chapter III we now have before us a
detailed model which we shall use in the next chapter to analyze the more dynamic element of the decision-making process and
the role of values in it.

NOTES

CHAPTER III

[1]For a recent presentation of the theory of value with an excellent bibliography, see Nicholas Rescher, *Introduction to Value Theory*, (Englewood Cliffs, N.J.: Prentice-Hall, Inc., 1969). Also see Stephen C. Pepper, "A Brief History of General Theory of Value," in *A History of Philosophical Systems*, ed. by Vergilius T. Ferm, (New York: Littlefield, 1950), pp. 493-503; Cornelius Kruse, "Western Theories of Value," in *Essays in East-West Philosophy*, ed. by C. A. Moore, (Honolulu: University of Hawaii Press, 1951), pp. 383-97; and J. Prescott Johnson, "The Fact Value Question in Early Modern Value Theory," *The Journal of Value Inquiry* I (1967), 64-71.

[2]Rescher, *Value Theory*, pp. 13-19.

[3]See, for example, Ethel M. Albert, "The Classification of Values: A Method and Illustration," *American Anthropologist* LVIII (1956), pp. 221-48; Stuart A. Dodd, "On Classifying Human Values," *American Sociological Review*, XVI (1951), pp. 645-65; Stephen C. Pepper, *The Sources of Value*, (Berkeley: University of California Press, 1958); Ralph Barton Perry, *Realms of Value: A Critique of Human Civilization*, (Westport, Conn.: Greenwood Press, Inc., 1954).

[4]Clyde Kluckhohn and others, "Values and Value-Orientations in the Theory of Action," in *Toward a General Theory of Action*, ed. by Talcott Parsons and Edward Shils, (New York: Harper and Row, 1951), p. 395.

[5]The authors which have been most helpful include Wolfgang Köhler, *The Place of Value in a World of Facts*, (New York: New American Library, 1966); Maurice Mandelbaum, *Phenomonology of Moral Experience*, (Baltimore: The Johns Hopkins Press, 1955); and Arthur J. Dyck, "A Gestalt Analysis of the Moral Data and Certain of Its Implications for Ethical Theory," (unpublished Ph.D. dissertation, Harvard University, 1965).

[6]Köhler, *The World of Values*, p. 36. See pp. 39, 65, 66, 69 and 70 for other examples of the ambiguous shifting of language.

[7]Mandelbaum, *Moral Experience*, p. 50.

[8]*Ibid.*

[9]Köhler, *The Place of Value*, p. 66. Köhler introduces this point as saying he will characterize requiredness. He uses the term 'interest' in the first two points then in the final point manages to include all the terms seemingly interchangeably, requiredness, valuation, interest and striving.

[10]*Ibid.*

113

[11]*Ibid.*, p. 67.

[12]Köhler, *The Place of Value*, p. 70.

[13]*Ibid.*, p. 86.

[14]*Ibid.*, pp. 73, 81, 86.

[15]Talcott Parsons, *Societies: Evolutionary and Comparative Perspectives*, (Englewood Cliffs, N.J.: Prentice-Hall, 1966), p. 28.

[16]Immanuel Kant, *Groundwork of the Metaphysic of Morals* (New York: Harper and Row, 1964), p. 82.

[17]Edward Westermarck, *Ethical Relativity* (Westport, Conn.: Greenwood Press, Inc., 1932).

[18]Susan C. Scrimshaw and Bernard Pasquariella, "Obstacles to Sterilization in One Community," *Family Planning Perspectives* II, No. 2 (October, 1970), pp. 40-42.

[19]William Graham Sumner, *Folkways: A Study of the Sociological Importance of Usages, Customs, Mores, and Morals* (New York: Dover, 1959).

[20]For a thorough discussion of the position of social relativism, see Karl Duncker, "Ethical Relativity," *Mind* XLVIII, 1939, pp. 39-56.

[21]Dyck, "A Gestalt Analysis," p. 39.

[22]*Ibid.*, p. 45.

[23]*Ibid.*, p. 48.

[24]*Ibid.*, p. 49.

[25]*Ibid.*, p. 51.

[26]C. Kluckhohn, "Values and Value-Orientations," pp. 388-433; Florence R. Kluckhohn and F. L. Strodtbeck, *Variations in Value Orientations* (Evanston, Ill.: Row, Peterson, 1961).

[27]C. Kluckhohn, "Values and Value-Orientations," p. 409.

[28]Paul Ramsey, *Deeds and Rules in Christian Ethics* (New York: Charles Scribner's Sons, 1967), p. 123.

[29]Parsons, "An Approach to the Sociology of Knowledge," pp. 141-42.

[30]Peter L. Berger, *The Sacred Canopy* (Garden City, New York: Doubleday, 1967), p. 181.

[31]Emile Durkheim, *The Elementary Forms of the Religious Life* (New York: The Free Press, 1965), p. 62.

[32] *Ibid.*, p. 53.

[33] Thomas Luckmann, *The Invisible Religion: The Problem of Religion in Modern Society*, (New York: The MacMillan Company, 1967), p. 43. We have already noted that Luckmann and Peter Berger with whom he developed his theory view reality as "socially constructed" or "objectivated" only in the sense that all symbol systems are products of culture. This should not be confused with the nominalist suggestion that there is no reality beyond the symbols.

[34] *Ibid.*, p. 53.

[35] *Ibid.*, p. 61.

[36] Paul Tillich, *Systematic Theology*, III (Chicago: The University of Chicago Press, 1963), p. 95.

[37] *Ibid.*, p. 98.

[38] *Ibid.*, p. 102.

[39] Paul Tillich, *Systematic Theology*, I (Chicago: The University of Chicago Press, 1963), p. 211.

[40] Luckmann, *Invisible Religion*, p. 61.

[41] *Ibid.*, p. 58.

[42] Parsons, "An Approach to the Sociology of Knowledge," p. 144.

[43] See Talcott Parsons, *The Social System* (New York: The Free Press, 1951), e.g., pp. 163-67, 367-83.

[44] Clyde Kluckhohn, "Values and Value-Orientations," p. 394.

[45] *Ibid.*, p. 409.

[46] Luckmann, *The Invisible Religion*, p. 57.

[47] Tillich, *Systematic Theory*, III, p. 95.

[48] *Ibid.*, p. 97.

CHAPTER IV

VALUE FACTORS IN SCIENTIFIC AND TECHNOLOGICAL DECISION-MAKING

Having developed a unified theory of scientific and technological action and analyzed the system of evaluation within
that system, we are at last ready to address ourselves to the
structure of the decision-making process itself and in particular the value factors in that decision-making process.

A. THE STRUCTURE OF DECISION-MAKING

Our first task will be to develop a model of the decision-
making process drawing on the model of the scientific and technological action system developed in the last two chapters.
There is a substantial literature on the theoretical aspects of
decision-making.[1] Space does not permit a thorough review of
this literature in the present discussion. What we shall present here is a rather elementary model of the components in the
process. First we shall construct a simple model, one which is
a first approximation to what goes on. Then we shall introduce
two types of complications.

1. *A Simplified Model.*

In Chapter III we developed the notion of the cultural
subsystem (i.e., the symbol system) as the locus of decision-
making (see Figure 4). Two elements of the cultural system
play the most direct role in the decision-making process.
These we termed cognitive and evaluative symbolization. Most
simplified it is through the interaction of empirical and evaluative ideas that a decision is reached which results in the
recommendation of an action. This interaction Parsons terms
the "value-science integrate." He sees it as the interaction
of scientific (empirical, cognitive) and evaluative components.
We feel this begs several questions, but believe we are dealing
with the same interaction process. We prefer to speak of these
dimensions as the primary factors in the decision-making process. What is extremely important--perhaps the most important
point to be made in this entire study--is that decision-making

117

requires of logical necessity both evaluative and (non-evaluative) factual elements.[2] It is not only practically, but logically impossible to make *any* decision scientifically in the sense of dealing solely with the "scientific (non-evaluative) facts."

The decision-making process, in this first simplified model, can be viewed as a syllogism in which the major premise is an evaluative one, one of the type "whenever conditions a, b, c exist one 'ought' (!) do thus and so." This major premise contains an evaluative term "ought." The minor premise contains the (non-evaluative) factual proposition obtained empirically through the methods available from the scientific disciplines. The form is: "Conditions a, b, c do exist." The logical conclusion can be deduced from the syllogism: "One ought to do thus and so." This, of course, is highly over-simplified, but is the basic structure of every so-called scientific or technological decision. It should be clear that the evaluative dimension is logically necessary.

The cultural system also contains the dimensions of expressive and existential meaning symbolization. It is obvious to any person with any knowledge of the human being as a social creature that these dimensions also play an important role in the decision-making process. In fact a cathexis for one's ethnic, religious, or class group may be the most important dimension in the decision-making process in terms of ability to predict a decision to be made. We shall term these factors the "secondary factors" not because they are necessarily of secondary importance, but because structurally they are usually indirectly incorporated into the process. It may be that one's being raised in and remaining loyal to the Roman Catholic Church is the most reliable predictor of decisions made regarding birth control. Nevertheless, this sociological fact of religious affiliation need not, and in a sophisticated presentation will not be included directly in the reasoning process leading to the decision. The major premise (the evaluative one) will be a statement of the conditions under which one *ought* not to practice birth control based on the cultural value complex regarding birth control. Now when one is asked to account for that statement, either sociologically or theologically, the cathexis of identification with the Catholic Church will be introduced, but it usually will not be incorporated directly. The same relationship exists with the symbolization for the grounding of meaning. The expressive and meaning ground dimensions are structurally the secondary factors feeding into the primary factors in the decision-making process. This structure is shown schematically in Figure 7.

2. *The Complications.*

Thus far we have presented an oversimplified model of the decision-making process. We shall now introduce some complications. We shall limit ourselves to two, each related to one of the primary factors. These both arise out of the observation of linguistic philosophers that language may be multifunctional.[3]

a. *Facts Will Be Evaluative.* Let us first examine the content of the minor premise, what has been variously termed the scientific, empirical, the (non-evaluative) facts. We have argued that a decision cannot logically be reached without combining this minor premise with the evaluative major premise. Now we shall have to blur these nice distinctions by arguing that, in two different ways, the minor premise may itself contain evaluative elements.

First, these are limits to what can be stated as "the facts." This selection takes place at many different levels--during one's education, specialization, and forgetting; more narrowly during the review of one's stored information when faced with a specific problem to be solved; and, perhaps most importantly, in the conceptualization of the problem. All of these require an evaluation for the purpose of selection. Even beyond this the process of observation is itself an evaluative one. When a scientist observes a scientific experiment or portion of nature, he first must select certain dimensions he considers significant. He must then choose a theoretical framework, his hypotheses, his methods of observation, the precision of his observation (two "significant" figures or five; a color roughly blue or one with precise wave length specified), the

PRIMARY FACTORS

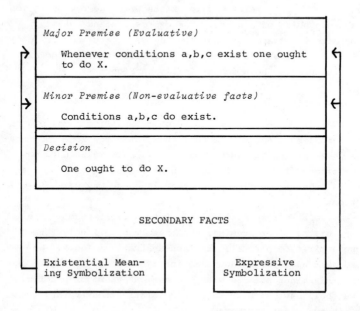

Fig. 7. Primary and Secondary Factors in Decision-Making

data worth recording and analyzing and reporting. Finally, at
the most elementary and often subconscious level choices are
made in the process of perception itself. The scientist who
thinks he has avoided the importation of values into these processes is naively mistaken. These are all choices, no matter
how simple, and, as we have argued, choice-making requires an
evaluative dimension. This is true at the steps of observation
and accumulation of the empirical facts which make up the substance of the minor premise itself. The points of value input
in the scientific process will be taken up in greater detail
later in this chapter.

There is a second way in which facts may be evaluative,
and here we are talking about something completely different.
It is common parlance among *homo scienticus* to speak of making
"scientific decisions." It is, in fact, true that often decisions are defended solely by stating (non-evaluative) empirically derived facts, for instance the following argument encountered in an interview the author conducted in research for
this study:

> Death rates from thromboembolism are three times
> as great among women using birth control pills
> than women who were normal controls. That is
> scientific proof that the pill should not be
> used.

This physician's argument contains only a statement of
empirically derivable fact and a conclusion which it is claimed
is scientific. We call the factual statement (which for our
purposes we may assume to be a sufficiently accurate report of
a reliable and generalizable study) in the above argument a
"value-loaded fact." The countervailing value-loaded fact
could be stated: "The death rate from not taking the pill including the risk of death resulting from predicted pregnancies
is higher than death rates from thromboembolisms when on the
pill." These two value-loaded facts each require suppressed
evaluative premises to complete the syllogisms. The general
form is one of assuming a value consensus in the evaluative
premise when it is suppressed. If questioned, however, one
must finally face and defend the evaluation being assumed. The
classical case, perhaps, is that of the compulsory blood

transfusion.[4] The seemingly scientific argument is that a blood transfusion must be given to a child because if it is not, according to the best scientific medical evidence, the child will die. The suppressed evaluation, of course, is that one ought always to give a blood transfusion under these conditions when a child will otherwise die. This premise is questioned not only by occasional religious objectors, but also by those who believe there are conditions where ethically a patient in extreme circumstances has a right to die. Recognition of the evaluative premise shifts the burden of the decision from beliefs about the medical facts of the situation where the physician clearly has expertise to the public judicial process where it is appropriate for evaluative judgments about such grave matters to be made.[5]

b. *Values May Be Factual*. Thus far when referring to the factual component (the minor premise) of the primary factors, we have hedged our terminology by the parenthetical statement that we were referring to the "non-evaluative" facts. Now we must face this question head on. Is there such a thing as a factual value? The view that values are totally separate from "the facts" is one, but only one, view. Here we must take up the debate we traced in the Introduction. We saw that on the one hand there were movements in history which tended to polarize the dichotomies between the scientific, the empirical, the non-evaluative and the religious, the vectorial, the evaluative. On the other hand there were movements which tended to see the points of contact between these two categories of phenomena holding that some evaluation may also be empirical.

We traced the discussion up to Descartes, Newton, and Locke who, we suggested, were the sources of the peculiarly modern phenomenon of the positivistic separation of fact and value. Newton's world was one devoid of ends and purposes. Locke makes a radical separation between primary and secondary qualities on the basis of whether there is anything like the ideas we have of the qualities existing in the bodies themselves:

> The ideas of primary qualities and their patterns
> do really exist in the bodies themselves; but the
> ideas, produced in us by these secondary qualities,

> have no resemblance of them at all. There is
> nothing like our ideas existing in the bodies
> themselves.[6]

This kind of distinction, as we shall see, laid the groundwork for the radical separation of the ethical, as a secondary quality having no "resemblance" in reality.

In contrast to Locke, Francis Hutcheson, a mid-eighteenth century ethicist argued for the close tie between ethical and other types of sensations. While he followed Locke in distinguishing primary and secondary qualities, he developed a "moral sense" theory in which ethics is put on an empirical perceptual basis closely paralleling the perceptions of the "external" senses. In his *Essay on the Nature and Conduct of the Passions and Affections, With Illustrations Upon the Moral Sense* he argues that moral sensations are received independently of our will according to the law of nature just as are sensations of extension and the like. The Author of Nature causes the correspondence of these sensations and the external "things of nature." In his *Introduction to Moral Philosophy*, Hutcheson maintains that by the moral sense "a certain course of action and plan of life is plainly recommended to us by nature....What is approved by this sense we count right and beautiful...."[7] While Newton was separating natural philosophy from moral philosophy Hutcheson saw them as inevitably linked into an integrated whole. His moral sense theory was a precursor to the empirical theory of Bentham and Mill.

G. E. Moore, in his *Principia Ethica*, developed Locke's distinctions drawing out their ethical implications. He argued that the notion of the "good" as the fundamental ethical quality was a simple, indefinable notion analogous to the simple notion, "yellow."[8] In Locke's terms it is a simple idea of the kind he called "secondary." We have argued that in history's ongoing struggle between the dichotomizers and the integrators, it is essential to know the context of the debate and the specific target of the argument. In Moore's case the target was Mill and the context was the claim that the good could be identified, i.e., defined, by empirically determining what is desired.[9] This view Moore, rightly or not, attributed to Mill. Moore claimed that any effort to define the good in terms of natural, empirically observable properties was a fallacy which he called the naturalistic fallacy.[10]

William Frankena has shown, however, that Moore's argument confuses several claims.[11] Most philosophers would grant that Moore is correct in attacking the notion that the good can be defined as the desired. The question, however, as Frankena points out, is not that one is attempting to define ethical characteristics in terms or non-ethical ones, nor even that one is attempting to define non-natural characteristics in terms of natural ones. The problem is a more generic one which Frankena calls the definist fallacy, i.e., "the process of confusing or identifying two properties, of defining one property by another, or of substituting one property for another."[12] While Moore has made his point in the context of the argument in which he is engaged--the good cannot be defined as the desired --this point in no way hinges upon the bifurcation of the natural and the non-natural, the ethical and the non-ethical, or the is and the ought. Whether or not ethical terms can be defined in terms of solely natural properties remains to be seen. Moore's subsuming of the good under the category of secondary qualities such as yellow gave rise to a school of ethical theory which pushed to its logical conclusion the claim that for secondary qualities there is nothing like our ideas existing in the bodies themselves. There is a direct historical and intellectual connection between Moore and the emotivists who go even beyond Moore to claim that ethical utterances are not only non-natural, as Moore claimed, they are not even cognitive statements at all.[13] They evince or express feelings and as such are not descriptive statements at all. Positivists, such as Ayer and Carnap, and emotivists such as Stevenson, to whom they are closely related, reject any possibility of verification of ethical claims. There is a radical dichotomy between the scientific descriptions and expressions of evaluative feelings. Since the days of Mill more plausible naturalistic analyses have been offered. The analyses of Firth[14] and Dyck[15] would be examples. Firth characterized his theory among other things as "objective" and "relational." Ethical statements are "objective" much in the way we used the term in Chapter III. They exist objectively in the phenomenal field independent of the

existence of the observer. The existence of this observer
around whom Firth constructs his analysis (the ideal observer)
is "logically irrelevant to truth or falsity of ethical statements."[16] His analysis is relational in the sense that it
claims ethical statements are asserting that a relationship
would exist between the acts or other things to which ethical
terms may be correctly applied and the ideal observer.[17] That
ethical statements are objective and relational directly challenges ethical analysis based upon the radical separation of
primary and secondary qualities. Ethical phenomena (acts or
other things) themselves possess properties which would tend to
produce the feeling of moral requiredness in the ideal observer.[18] To make such analysis requires the collapsing of the
radical distinction between the primary and secondary qualities
of objects or events.

The foregoing discussion should demonstrate that it is by
no means clear that ethical claims can be radically separated
from those of fact. The same type of arguments can be offered
for the other types of objectively localized evaluation we presented in Chapter III. Whether or not one maintains that objectively localized evaluative claims are statements of a particular type of fact or expressions of emotions, feelings, and
prescriptions makes a tremendous difference when one wants to
go about resolving disputes about these evaluative claims. For
our purposes, what is important, however, is that even if ethical and other objectively localized evaluative claims are seen
as claims about a particular type of fact, the evaluative propositions which constitute one of the primary factors in the
structure of decision-making are still independent from the
non-evaluative facts which constitute the other of the primary
factors. According to the emotivists the major premise of the
syllogism is a prescription, an evinced feeling in principle
not capable of verification. According to the naturalists, it
is a cognitive statement which may contain factual elements,
i.e., statements about ethical and other evaluative facts, in
principle capable of empirical verification, but not--and this
is critical--not by the technique of the discipline which would
be responsible for verifying the facts of the minor premise.
In either case, however, the source of the primary factor we

have identified as the major premise of the decision-making syllogism is independent of the particular scientific discipline from which the non-evaluative empirical facts are drawn which constitute the minor premise. This means that values must of necessity be incorporated into every decision which requires data from the scientific enterprise. In the next section of this chapter we shall attempt to develop a classification of the points at which these values enter the scientific and technological process.

B. VALUE FACTORS IN SCIENCE AND TECHNOLOGY

In the arguments about the possibility of a value-free science many different types of value inputs are discussed. Even the strongest advocate of value-freedom in science is willing to recognize certain types of value inputs while the most radical polemicists allow the necessity of controls on value expression in some aspects of the scientific enterprise. We shall now present, in brief summary form, a cybernetic model of the types of value inputs in scientific and technological action. We have abstracted three stages at which values play a part. They are represented in Figure 8.

After describing each stage and the value factors associated with that stage, we shall describe the characteristic error which arises from failing to take into account the value inputs at that stage.

1. *The Pre-scientific Stage (Type I Value Factors).*

Read Bain, in a 1939 statement of editorial policy for the *American Sociological Review*, states that:

> He (the scientist) is influenced by non-scientific values in his selection of research problems, but once the problem is selected, he must banish as completely as possible all pre-dispositions, wishes, practical considerations, personal preferences, and value judgments except those implicit in scientific method.[19]

It is clear that Bain, in his orthodox statement of the value-free science position, recognizes the necessity and significance of value inputs in pre-scientific selection of

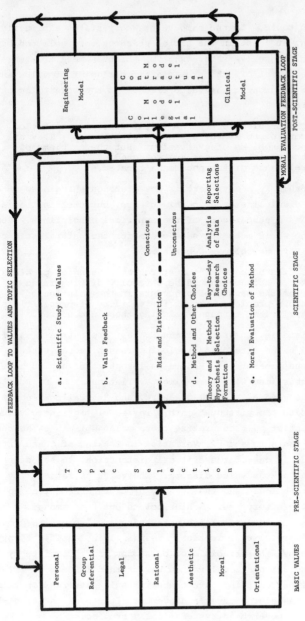

Fig. 8. Cybernetic Model Showing Types of Value Factors in the System of Science and Technology

research topic. In the same vein, Weber states explicitly that
problems, at least in the social sciences, are selected by the
value-relevance (*Wertbeziehung*) of the phenomena treated. He
attempts to set off the pre-scientific element of value input
in order to protect the value freedom of the scientific enterprise itself:

> The problems of the empirical disciplines are, of
> course, to be solved "non-evaluatively." They are
> not problems of evaluation. But the problems of
> the social sciences are selected by the value-
> relevance of the phenomena treated.[20]

Presumably, Weber here is not distinguishing between empirical disciplines and social science, but treating social
science as a subcategory of the empirical disciplines. Certainly he would make the same claim for the natural sciences.
Talcott Parsons follows Weber here.

> ...the bases of interest for the posing of problems
> for a science should be carefully distinguished
> from the canons of procedure in the solution of
> those problems, and of the validity of propositions
> arrived at through following those procedures.[21]

Aristotle, in *Nichomachean Ethics*, presents a list of generalized value categories including reason, moral virtue,
honor, and pleasure.[22] Modern philosophers of ethics have accepted this list with some slight variations. W. D. Ross includes knowledge, virtue, pleasure, and "the allocation of
pleasure to the virtuous" in his review of "intrinsic value."[23]
The scientist *must* concretize these value options as he chooses
what he wants to study. Variation in ranking of these intrinsic goods is one of the critical distinctions in scientists'
positions of the value dispute. The value of rationality associated with logic and the pursuit of truth are central to the
scientific enterprise. Köhler points out that among the values
essential to the scientific enterprise are "objective procedure," "careful verification," "genuinely scientific theory,"
and perhaps "the principle of parsimony" and "consistency."[24]
Among the orientational values we outlined in Chapter III,
there almost certainly are characteristic patterns for the sci-
entist--man over nature, achievement, future orientation--but
these have never been systematically studied.

On the other hand there are values which are not emphasized by scientists, or at least by many scientists--aesthetic experience, sometimes pleasure, and moral values such as justice. These characteristic value patterns will influence from the beginning the types of problems a scientist chooses to study as well as the way his investigation is carried out. It should also be obvious that social actors other than the scientist such as the funding agency or research institution can play a key role in providing specific options for concretizing intrinsic goods. Participants in the *Werturteilsstreit* differ greatly on the importance they assign to the value inputs of the pre-scientific stage.

Although even the scientists we called "pure scientists" in Chapter I concede the importance of values in the selection of research topics, they frequently argue that this is of little importance because, provided the investigation is carried out following the rules of empirical science and without the incorporation of values into investigation itself, the results of the study should be the same regardless of what the original motive or values were which led the scientist to the investigation in the first place.[25]

There are two problems with this argument. The first is, of course, that scientists do not, in fact, carry out their work in exact conformity to the ideal of scientific value neutrality. (We shall discuss this in our next section when we take up the scientific stage.) Secondly, even if they could carry out the work that they do in accordance with the ideal of neutrality, pre-scientific value inputs would still determine exactly what they choose to investigate and what they choose to leave unknown. If some facts are "value loaded" in that they would, when coupled with generally agreed upon value premises, lead to certain conclusions, it is quite possible that scientists will consciously or unconsciously choose research topics which will produce "value-loaded" facts supporting their values while countervailing "value-loaded" facts will go undiscovered. The scientists who become experts in any given area enter that area on the basis of a particular set of values. They differ from the rest of humanity in that they see this area as the one

area which, for one reason or another, is more important to
them than any other. This means that they stand in a very peculiar relationship to the topic they have chosen to study.
They see it in a way that no one else does.

If the "experts" on any given topic stand in a peculiar
relationship to it, then it stands to reason that the consensus
of experts also may be systematically skewed by this peculiar
value perspective. For this reason we call overlooking the importance of pre-scientific value inputs the "fallacy of the
consensus of experts." Whenever one hears reference to the
consensus of experts as the authority for an empirical statement it is always essential to ask if the consensus of those
experts has been affected by the peculiar value consensus of
those experts. This is particularly obvious in politically
sensitive areas. Most would see the fallacy of determining
policy on whether to drop an atomic bomb on an enemy city by
asking for the consensus of military generals or atomic bomb
physicists. Not only do they have no particular expertise on
the evaluative component in the decision-making process (the
major premise in our discussion earlier in this chapter), in a
case such as this it is quite possible that those who have
chosen careers as military generals or atomic bomb physicists
may have systematic value biases about bombing enemy cities.

Even if we could assume that biases in the reading of the
scientific data are excluded from the consensus of the experts,
the consensus still may be influenced by the particular set of
values of the experts with regard to the kinds of observations
they have chosen to make and the certainty they demand for
their conclusions. We shall illustrate this and some other
types of value factors by referring to controversy currently
raging in the medical profession over the use of tolbutamide,
a drug given orally for certain kinds of mild diabetes. A
group of researchers, calling themselves the University Group
Diabetes Program (UGDP), on the basis of their study of the
compound, concluded that diet control plus tolbutamide was no
more effective than diet alone in prolonging life among mild,
adult-onset diabetics and may be less effective than diet alone
or diet plus insulin in preventing cardiovascular deaths.[26]

The Food and Drug Administration, the American Diabetes Association and the AMA's Council on Drugs all endorsed the study
and the FDA issued a statement saying that oral hypoglycemic
agents were recommended only in cases "which cannot be controlled by diet alone and for whom insulin is unacceptable or im-
practical."

The study was clearly a complicated and controversial one.
There were questions of methodology and conclusions which were
open to debate. The situation was one of great uncertainty
about the use of tolbutamide. The result was that a group of
thirty-four noted diabetologists issued a statement attacking
the FDA recommendation and charging that it compromised the
physician's freedom to prescribe.[27] Dr. Robert Bradley claimed
that the statement represented "the majority opinion of practicing diabetologists." FDA Commissioner Charles Edwards countered by claiming that there appeared to be a consensus favoring support of the conclusions. For our purposes the interesting thing is that both men appealed to the consensus of medical
experts to buttress their argument. What was at stake here was
whether or not a therapeutic treatment should be used when
there was uncertainty about its effectiveness and safety. Both
sides assumed that the experts' consensus would have settled
the issue. We would argue that what is at stake here is not a
technical question at all, but who should make decisions about
what to do when there is uncertainty. If there is a peculiar
value perspective among the experts--one which says that when
in doubt one should continue the procedure or one which sees
the freedom of the physician to prescribe as crucial--then even
the consensus of the experts must be questioned. If the consensus of diabetes experts is that when there is uncertainty
the drug should be used, but the legitimate public authority
(in this case the FDA) brings to bear a different value orientation, we cannot see why the medical experts' consensus should
take precedence.

2. *The Scientific Stage (Type II Value Factors)*.

The diagram in Figure 8 indicates that after decisions are
made regarding selection of research topic, the scientific

enterprise moves to what we have called the scientific stage.
It is at this stage along with the third or technological stage
that the most heat has been generated in the *Werturteilsstreit*.

In Chapter I we noted that in 1904 Weber, along with
Werner Sombart and Edgar Jaffe, assumed the editorship of the
Archiv für Sozialwissenschaft und Sozialpolitik. Weber's essay
on "'Objectivity' in Social Science and Social Policy" states
the classical position of the pure scientist about the necessity of value-freedom at the scientific stage:

> In the pages of this journal, especially in the
> discussion of legislation, there will inevitably
> be found social *policy*, i.e., the statement of
> ideals, in addition to social *science*, i.e., the
> analysis of facts. But we do not by any means
> intend to present such discussions as "science"
> and we will guard as best we can against allowing
> these two to be confused with each other....In
> other words, it should be made explicit just where
> the arguments are addressed to the analytical
> understanding and where to the sentiments.[28]

At the scientific stage we have identified at least five
types of value inputs. Holders of varying positions in the
value-dispute will treat these value inputs in different ways.
We shall merely present in summary form the value factors of
the scientific stage.

a. *The Scientific Study of Values (Type IIa)*. While the
positivist philosophical tradition, at least in its extreme
forms, argues for the utter separation of fact and value, the
pure scientist recognizes that values are a valid subject for
scientific study. In his paper on "The Meaning of 'Ethical
Neutrality' in Sociology and Economics," which grew out of the
Werturteilsstreit of the Verein für Sozialpolitik, Weber argues:

> What is really at issue is the intrinsically simple
> demand that the investigator and teacher should
> keep unconditionally separate the establishment of
> empirical facts (including the "value-oriented"
> conduct of the empirical individual whom he is in-
> vestigating) and *his* own practical evaluations,
> i.e., his evaluation of these facts as satisfactory
> or unsatisfactory (including among these facts
> evaluations made by the empirical persons who are
> the objects of investigation.)[29]

Even while Weber is defending the wall of the fact-value dualism, however, he makes perfectly clear that, as the parentheses

in the above quotation reveal, values may properly be the object of scientific study. He argues that an "almost inconceivable misunderstanding which constantly recurs is that the propositions which I propose imply that empirical science cannot treat 'subjective' evaluations as the subject-matter of its analysis...."[30]

It should be clear that this concession to the attackers of the fact-value dichotomy need not challenge the ideal of scientific value-freedom. Dahrendorf has called this value factor within the scientific stage one of the "pseudo-problems" regarding value-free social science.[31]

b. *Value Feedback From the Scientific Enterprise (Type IIb)*. A second value factor in the scientific stage may also be termed a "pseudo-problem." It is diagrammed as a feedback loop in our cybernetic model. We are beginning to recognize the at least partial validity of what the Marxists have been saying. Substructural factors including science and technology have profound effects on our systems of value. Dramatic changes in the moral evaluation of birth control in the last fifteen years almost certainly are related to technological breakthroughs in this area.

Herbert Marcuse warns of the dehumanizing effects of science and technology when they become political. Science and technology in their political form restructure the means of production, social aspirations, and personal relationships. They contribute to the creation of a "new society,"[32] what Marcuse calls the "society of total mobilization." One of the most explicit analyses of this relationship is Theodore J. Gordon's article "The Feedback Between Technology and Values."[33] Emmanuel Mesthane and others in the Program on Technology and Society at Harvard are also deeply interested in this issue.

Most feedback involves "technology" or the application of scientific methods and information for the solving of human problems. This is what we have termed the third or application stage of our diagram. A feedback loop will be seen connecting the application stage to the values which affect pre-scientific selection. We feel, however, that there is also a feedback from the scientific stage itself to the basic values in the

system. The existence of the scientific enterprise itself has
enhanced our evaluation of Truth ("for Truth's sake"). It
modifies our entire world perspective shifting man's relationship to nature, man, and the gods. At a more concrete level
our confidence in the scientific enterprise probably accounts
for apathy toward environmental pollution and geriatric ill-
nesses.

This feedback from the scientific enterprise we have identified as a second value factor at this stage. Within this
stage we maintain that this also is a "pseudo-problem." While
feedback may have tremendous consequences for our values and
through this affect the pre-scientific selection of research
topics, it does not directly challenge the ideal of value-freedom *within the scientific stage*. We shall have to look to
other factors at this level before this norm is challenged more
directly.

c. *Bias and Distortion (Type IIc)*. If elementary school
teachers are led to believe that certain students in their
classes can be expected, "based on scientific tests" to show a
large increase in their academic performance, such an increase
is likely to come about.[34] In a pharmacology laboratory the
standard test for the effectiveness of analgesics and narcotics
is to observe the pain response of a mouse or other animal.
This is usually measured by the flick of the tail or the lift-
ing of the foot. Having observed competent pharmacologists
administer this test to thousands of perpetually squirming
mice, the author has come to doubt the objectivity of many of
these tests. We suspect we were observing a sophisticated version of the placebo effect. These effects are magnified as the
observations become more subjective and ambiguous. In the discipline of anthropology two anthropologists have upon occasion
studied the same community at presumably comparable times and
found contradictory characteristics. In the field of sociology
interviewing and coding present highly ambiguous situations
where experimenter value inputs can frequently produce grave
biases and distortion. Robert Rosenthal deserves much of the
credit for bringing to the foreground the pervasiveness of this
value input.[35]

We are using bias and distortion in our discussion to refer to the systematic modification of scientific observations
and procedures as a function of the researcher's particularistic value preferences. We shall reserve to the next section
our discussion of value inputs into method selection and reporting. Within the limits of modifications which take place
when there is a deviation in the data recorded from the thing
observed or a deviation from the specified procedure, we find
it necessary to distinguish two types of bias and distortion
based on whether or not the modification is conscious. While
conscious and unconscious modification of data and procedures
have much in common (most significantly they are both examples
of deviation from the ultimate scientific norm of "objectivity"), they also have several important distinguishing characteristics. Conscious manipulation of procedures and data to get
desired results is clearly recognized as dishonest, scientifically invalid, and without excuse. This kind of biasing of
scientific work is, of course, ultimately self-defeating if the
goal is either scientific value of truth or the solution of
specific technological or social problems. It can occur, however, when other values--personal gain, the need to publish a
consistent paper or the need to satisfy the funder of the re-
search--become dominant. We believe that although instances of
this out-and-out conscious biasing of scientific work are reported they are very rare. Unconscious bias and distortion, on
the other hand, is accepted as pervasively inevitable, even if
wrong. In the tolbutamide controversy charges have been made
that the interests of the drug companies may have influenced
the views of some of those participating in the debate. While
the evidence for this is doubtful, it cannot be denied that
many of the participants in the controversy have very deep
vested interests in various aspects of diabetes research and in
their roles as government agents. While unconscious biasing
from interests such as these will be opposed by any honest scientist, he will also grant that total elimination of these
value inputs is impossible. The methods of control of conscious and unconscious distortion must be quite different as
are the evaluations of the two types of offenders of the

value-free norm. While the former is immoral and unforgive-
able, the latter is looked upon as incompetent and careless.

In contrast to the first two value factors in the scientific stage, which were labeled "pseudo-problems," the value
inputs in bias and distortion of procedure and data recording
are truly inputs. They lie at the base of the ideal of scientific value-freedom. Even the most radical challengers of the
ideal must be reluctant to abandon the norm of value-freedom
when this type of value factor is involved.

d. *Method and Other Choices Within the Scientific Stage
(Type IId)*. So far within the scientific stage we have isolated two value factors which we have labeled "pseudo-problems"
and now one value input which most participants in the *Werturteilsstreit* agree should ideally be eliminated. It is extremely important to separate the modification and manipulation of
experimental procedures and recording and reporting of data
from a further value input into the scientific stage, the making of method and other choices. We have thus far recognized
that selection of topics for scientific investigation requires
value inputs. Most people, upon reflection, will also grant
that applying scientific information to the solving of human
problems requires value inputs. This we shall discuss below in
our discussion of what we have termed the application or post-
scientific stage. The problem of method and other choices
within the scientific stage frequently goes unnoticed, however.
This is in our opinion the most critical factor in the dispute
over value-freedom in the sciences. It is extremely important
that these be separated from biasing and distorting execution
of chosen methods and recording and reporting of data as discussed above.

We demonstrated in the first section of this chapter that
every decision requires a value input. This is often recognized for the pre- and post-scientific stages, but applies
equally to the scientific stage itself. Decisions or choices
must be made at every step in the scientific enterprise. Some
of the early and major ones are sometimes collapsed into the
pre-scientific stage, some of the later ones into the post-
scientific stage. But we would maintain that choices are made

at every step of what is commonly recognized as scientific endeavor. If this is so it becomes unfeasible to speak of
"value-free science." We shall attempt to illustrate this per-
vasive interpenetration of (value-based) choices and scientific
observation by pointing out five steps in the scientific stage
and the choices made in each step.

(1) The first step in scientific inquiry which we shall
discuss is theory selection and hypothesis formation. Dahrendorf argues that hypothesis formation, much like topic selection, requries value inputs, but that this does not jeopardize
scientific objectivity because

> neither the values nor the thought processes of
> a scientist determine the validity of his hypo-
> theses; their validity is determined only by
> empirical test.[36]

There is a certain validity in Dahrendorf's point. It requires,
of course, that ideological bias and distortion of the empirical test be considered as a separate problem, but Dahrendorf is
aware of this. Dahrendorf thus reaches a conclusion similar to
Weber's on this point by separating the functions of hypothesis
formation and hypothesis testing.[37]

This movement, however, minimizes the interaction between
theory formation and empirical testing. Boguslaw, in a discussion of the theoretical perspectives in systems analysis, has
shown how closely concrete empirical analyses are related to
the theoretical model of the analyst.[38] Merton argues that empirical testing is a critical factor in the formation of theory.[39] If theory and empirical observation are so closely connected, it becomes difficult to maintain, as Dahrendorf does,
that hypothesis formation is a "pseudo-problem." This interaction is not primarily from ideological bias and distortion,
but from choices made in the later steps of the scientific
stage. A Marxist and Freudian differ not only in their theories about social problems, but also in the methodology of
testing hypotheses.

Probably the most clearly recognized influence of theory
selection on scientific study is the necessary adoption of a
theoretical framework for social scientific study. Integration

or balancing theories often lead to very different methods and conclusions from conflict or dissonance theories. In our first footnote in Chapter II we discussed the problem of theory selection with regard to the present analysis of scientific decision-making. We warned against the assumption that combining two or more theories would present the "total" or "unbiased" analysis. Burch has shown the importance of theory for the scientific study of religion.[40] Friedrichs has reviewed more generally the importance of theory in sociology.[41] Theory also influences the analysis of the natural sciences. Kim has shown that theory influences the explanation of adoption and diffusion of an innovation applied to the intra-uterine contraceptive device.[42] Working in pharmacology laboratories we found that the theory of drug action was the major if not sole determinant of the types of experimentation carried out.

(2) A second step in the scientific stage which requires value inputs is the choice of methods for testing hypotheses. Walton, in a review of community power studies done by sociologists and political scientists, has shown that conclusions reached were heavily dependent upon methods of study selected which, in turn, were dependent upon the discipline of the researcher.[43] He also suggests that the researcher, or more accurately the researcher's values, are related to the selection of discipline. Record, among others, has demonstrated how the socialization process for the young academician in his academic training and in his "research apprenticeship" subtly and subconsciously forms the value structure as well as the live method options open to the researcher.[44]

The fact that in retrospect method choices in community power studies are shown to be operationalizing two somewhat different conceptions of power is of secondary importance. For many years social scientists and the lay readers of their material were unaware of the value inputs in these method choices. Suggestions that the two major methods be combined to get the "true picture" of community power reveal that many still do not grasp the significance of these value inputs.

In the tolbutamide debate we have been discussing, conflict over choice of methods for the research has played a major role in the controversy. The study out of which the controversy developed was a retrospective one. Some of the signers of the statement opposing the FDA position have argued that retrospective studies do not give a clear indication of the efficacy of the drug because the population is a selected one. The critics of the study of the UGDP also charged that the study used a fixed dose of tolbutamide while different results might have been obtained by tailoring the dose to the individual patient's needs. Finally Drs. Bradley and Seltzer pointed out that the death rates due to tolbutamide appeared to be leveling off near the end of the study. They argue that if the study had been continued different conclusions might have been drawn. Again the choice of end point for a set of observations is a choice that has to be made. If it is done consciously to manipulate data we have a case of bias and distortion of the type discussed above, but *some* choice must be made and it must be made on the basis of a set of evaluations.

(3) Even if we consider that major method selections as well as hypothesis formation are "pre-scientific" in character, we still must face a third step where choices must be made and values must be expressed. We are referring to the infinite number of day-to-day choices that the scientist *must* make even after he has selected his basic methods. One of these is the role or image of the investigator. Doing research on race in South Africa, van den Berghe found that he *had* to decide whether to behave as most white South Africans did or to act in a "color-blind" fashion which reflected his own value preferences.[45] Madan comments on the necessity of the Indian sociologist to be identified by caste (or to take on the even more decisive image of ignoring caste).[46] Similar role choices must be made by all scientists. For our purposes the important thing is that some choice must be made.

Value inputs penetrate even more deeply than role selection. Choice of sample location, sample size, and sample characteristics are probably more critical than is often realized.[47] The extent and quality of controls in experimentation must also be decided. In the tolbutamide case the critics suggested that some unaccounted-for factor may have caused some of the deaths particularly in certain of the clinics in the study. The choice of variables worth (N.B.) controlling is one that must be made in the selection of research design for any scientific study.

One of the most critical of the routine choices made in this third stage is which data are to be observed and recorded. Even unconsciously the potential perceptual field is evaluated so that only "significant" portions are perceived. From what is perceived only a small portion is actually recorded. It is impossible as well as useless to try to record all that is observed. Selection must be on the basis of what is considered valuable. All of these day-to-day decisions which the scientist must make indicate that it is fruitless to try to separate all value inputs into the pre- and post-scientific stages.

(4) The fourth step in the scientific stage which requires choice, and therefore value inputs, is the analysis of data. Such choices as the types of statistics and the significance levels used should be included here. We have seen that one of the critical questions in the tolbutamide controversy is how certain a conclusion must be before it is "certain enough." Is something established as a fact when the confidence level is ninety-five percent or must it be 99.9 percent? Dr. Byron W. Brown, a statistician supporting the UGDP study, argues that paired subgroup comparisons is a valid way of comparing groups in the study. But Dr. Stanley Schor argues that looking at the same statistics another way suggests a different conclusion. The use of differing statistical tests, as often can happen, produces different implications. The choices made play a critical role.

(5) Finally, the fifth step in the scientific stage is the selection of material for reporting. The researcher must decide what he considers of such significance that it should be reported. Every researcher must face, consciously or unconsciously, the dilemma reported by Richard Brymer and Buford Farris:

> Although we have tried to select the *relevant characteristics* for the composite cases, the fact remains that we have still presented some data and not others. The logical possibility exists that we have failed to present the very data which are needed by other scientists.[48]

e. *Moral Evaluation of Scientific Methods (Type IIe).*
There remains one final value factor which impinges on the scientific enterprise itself. That is the moral evaluation of the
research procedure. This aspect has received much attention of
late, and we can only mention it in passing. Kelman's volume
treats this area in detail.[49] His work suggests that there are
at least two separate components to this moral evaluation.
First, research procedures can and must be morally evaluated in
themselves. Some of the major ethical issues at stake here include privacy, informed consent and deception, psychic or physical harm to the subject, and respect for the subject whether
it is an individual or a group.[50] This aspect of moral evaluation of research is sometimes formulated as a conflict between
the norms of science and other social obligations.[51] Naive,
even deceived, subjects are perhaps acceptable or even required
from the standpoint of scientific procedure, but questionable
on non-scientific grounds. Our tolbutamide case also has an
important value input at this level. Many of the questions
raised could theoretically be settled by repeating the experiment. If the study had been continued for a longer period we
would have known if the death rates from tolbutamide did indeed
level off. The problem arises, however, because the experiment
was discontinued because of an essentially moral judgment. The
UGDP investigators, alarmed by the incidence of cardiovascular
deaths in the tolbutamide group agreed to discontinue tolbutamide therapy in October of 1969. Dr. Bradley, spokesman for
the critics, called this a "disastrous mistake." Here is a
clear case of an ethical judgment about the experimental procedure which could not be avoided. Dr. Bradley's position reflects a different set of values (a set which we suggested may
be related to entry into a scientific career in the first
place). Evidently he placed higher value on the knowledge
which would have been gained by continuing the experiment than
on the lives of the subjects which would have been placed in
jeopardy by continuing. This may or may not have been a case
of ethical indifference. He may have made the ethical judgment, right or wrong, that in the long run more people would
benefit by continuing the study. One cannot escape the fact,

however, that an ethical decision had to be made. Whether he decided that Truth was more valuable than what was moral or he decided that the good of the many was ethically dominant over the good of the few who were subjects, Dr. Bradley made an ethical decision just as those who stopped the experiment did.

A second component of moral evaluation of scientific procedure is suggested by Kelman's discussion of "The Social Scientist as Producer of Social Forces."[52] The researcher can and does envision anticipated uses for his findings. Most scientists are willing to admit that they have some responsibility for anticipated uses, although there is considerable disagreement on the extent. This suggests a feedback loop between the post-scientific or application stage and the scientific stage. This is represented in our diagram in Figure 8.

We have called the overlooking of the importance of pre-scientific value inputs "the fallacy of consensus of expert opinion." Problems also arise from overlooking the value inputs in the scientific stage. There is a lingering ideal of the scientist, in his scientific role, as "value-free." We shall call the overlooking of the value inputs of the scientific stage "the fallacy of the ideal type." In fact there are two prongs to this fallacy. The first arises out of the value inputs from bias and distortion. Often biases and distortion that exist in the real, less than perfect world are overlooked. Behaving as if value-free ideal type were being achieved is the first prong of the fallacy of the ideal type.

In addition to value inputs in the scientific stage from bias and distortion we described value inputs from method and other choices and value inputs from moral evaluation of scientific procedures. We have argued throughout this chapter that these value inputs cannot, in principle, be eliminated even ideally. Behaving as if the value-free ideal type *could* be achieved in this sense is the second prong of the fallacy of the ideal type.

From this a provocative question arises. If it is fallacious to assume that the ideal is ever reached in practice with respect to bias and distortion or could be reached even in principle with respect to method and other choices and moral evaluation of methods, then maybe a new ideal itself is called for. An analogy from Troeltsch is suggested. He distinguished between an ideal of absolute natural law held by the Stoics to be applicable to man in the pristine state before the fall and a relative natural law for man after the fall, no less ideal, but ideal for man in a different condition.[53] Is it not possible that in the light of the shortcomings in the ideal of the value-free scientist pointed out by the first and second fallacies of the ideal type, a new ideal is called for--one which would take account of the fallenness of *homo scienticus* so that he never can eliminate bias and distortion although he must ever continue in his effort and one which also would take into account the impossibility of eliminating value inputs in method choices and moral evaluation of methods? The construction of a new ideal type for scientific man cannot be undertaken here, but we suggest that it is a worthwhile project for the future.

This completes our discussion of the scientific stage and leads us to our analysis of the value factors in the application of scientific information to the solving of human problems, the third and final stage of our discussion.

3. *The Post-scientific or Application Stage (Type III Value Factors).*

Technology we have defined as the systematic application of scientific methods and knowledge for the solving of human problems. All application requires decision-making and hence, as we have shown in the first part of this chapter, requires value inputs. The scientist is at this point placed in an inherently contradictory position. As scientist he has particular expertise in the non-evaluative, cognitive information necessary for the minor premise of the decision-making procedure. As scientist, however, he has no peculiar expertise in the value choices, ethical and otherwise, which are required for the evaluative factor which is the major premise. In Chapter II we argued that the scientist's cognitive, descriptive task was universalistic in the sense that it was not "filtered through" his system of meaning, value, and cathexis. When we come to the application stage, however, there *must* be an evaluative factor. It is, by definition, impossible for this to be universalistic in the sense we have described. The problem is thus seen as one where the technical expert is the only one with expertise in one of the factors, but, at the same time, has no peculiar expertise in the evaluative factor.

Often the technical expert is consciously or unconsciously assumed to have such expertise. Obstetricians, trained in the physiology and pathology of the uterus, are placed on abortion panels in hospitals throughout the country; yet the strictly technical side of an abortion, barring special cases, is the one element where little disagreement is likely to arise. This tendency to grant those with expertise in the technical issues on a given question expertise in the evaluation and decision-making functions we have termed the fallacy of generalization of expertise. It is the process of granting expertise in the sphere of evaluative symbolization to those who have recognized expertise in the area of (non-evaluative) cognitive symbolization. "Pure scientists" are aware of this and sound the call for a hasty retreat behind the walls of value-free science.

There are two difficulties with this solution, however. First, we have already shown that value-based choices penetrate so far into the enclave of the scientific stage that separation of a value-free retreat becomes meaningless. Second, upon reflection it seems that almost all scientific endeavor has a technological, clinical, or other applied science component to it. This is apparent for the fields of clinical medicine and psychology as well as engineering, but is equally true for any efforts to apply science to the solving of human problems. There are even elements of envisioned potential application of what at first seems to be pure pursuit of "truth for truth's sake." Funders of research almost always provide funds as a means of solving problems of interest to them. In the case of university and governmentally funded research the envisioned application may be relatively long run, but most "pure scientists" are quick to defend themselves against the charge that their work is utterly without potential use.[54]

The real issue arises not in the scientist separating himself from any value inputs, but in the relation of the scientist's own personal values to the values of the layman in the action system. Our diagram in Figure 8 presents four models for this relationship in the application stage. We have assigned names to these four models, the clinical, engineering, and collegial, and the contractual, not to suggest that the, clinical relationship, for instance, must show the characteristics we describe here, but that these professional roles have tendencies inherent in them which lead to the value relationships of the type we describe.

a. *The Clinical Model*. Our first model is based on the value relationships between the clinician as the professional actor and the patient as the lay actor. The layman consults the professional such as a physician because he is generally aware of distress in the organic sector and wants advice about his problem. The physician is expected to "prescribe" a solution. The nature of the situation is such that the patient's values at best are only partially taken into account. In the clinical model the professional usually has higher status than the layman. The relationship is often characterized by appeals for advice in the value as well as the technical sphere. The physician, as proto-typical example of the clinician, often assumes the role of generalized authority figure. Through the fallacy of generalization of expertise the patient is even often willing to grant him this role. The literature of the professional role, as we discussed in Chapter II, characterizes the physician as parent or priest. Robert Wilson likens the doctor's office to a sanctuary; the physician is "removed from the prosaic and mundane," regarded by the patient (according to Wilson) as "a substance unlike himself."[55] One physician with delusions of grandeur in the direction of generalization of his expertise has claimed in a conversation with the author that "every patient is a dependent child who demands of his physician that he be a good parent."

In the tolbutamide debate the participants in both sides of the discussion assumed that the technical experts were the proper authorities to be making the decisions. If we are correct in claiming that the real issue in the policy decision required at the moment is what one must do in the light of great uncertainty, we have a problem which is essentially one of what orientational and other values are to be incorporated into the major premise. Under conditions of uncertainty does one continue tolbutamide or not? Further research may eliminate some of the uncertainty, but, unless we are wrong, no amount of medical research or technical expertise can tell us what is the *right* thing to do when we have uncertainty. To assume that the experts can solve this question is a generalization of authority which is uncalled for. In any case it is impossible for the clinician to consult his patient seeking the latter's value input for every decision made. The result is often an over-valuing of the professional's values at the expense of the layman's. We have a generalization of expertise.

The professor-student relationship has much in common with the clinical situation. The status relationship is similar. The student often turns to the professor for advice in value spheres or at least for recommendations for reading the reflection. Weber was extremely critical of excesses of professorial value inputs in the teaching sphere saying that:

> Of all the types of prophecy, this "personally" tinted professorial type of prophecy is the only one which is altogether repugnant. An unprecedented situation exists when a large number of officially accredited prophets do their preaching not on the streets, or in churches or other public places or in sectarian conventicles, but rather feel themselves competent to enunciate their evaluations on ultimate questions "in the name of science" in governmentally privileged lecture halls in which they are neither controlled, checked by discussion, nor subject to contradiction.[56]

b. *The Engineering Model*. Our second model arises out of an attempt to correct the difficulties of the first. Whereas the clinical model tends toward over-evaluation of the technical expert's own values at the expense of the lower status, poorly informed layman, the engineering model tends toward under-evaluation of the significance of the technical expert's values in deference to relatively high status, layman employers. In contrast to clinical "practice," much of what is generally termed "applied science," social as well as physical and biological, tends to have the characteristics of the engineering model.

In its most extreme form the applied scientist acting in the engineering model can become a moral imbecile selling his services to the highest bidder, without consideration of the moral implications of the work he is doing. In our diagram we indicate that the engineering model (speaking of the ideal case) lacks a feedback loop to the scientific stage so that scientific research is completely divorced from the potential uses of the work. Project Camelot demonstrated tendencies toward the engineering model, but the fact that eventually sociologists as well as Latin American politicians began to question the possible uses of the research indicates that social scientists are able to overcome the "I'm only doing my job" . mentality which characterizes lack of value inputs by the scientist to the application stage.[57]

The fact that both over-emphasis and under-emphasis on the values of the technical expert occurs in the application stage gives rise to interesting and perplexing difficulties. We shall show that Weber was contending against both tendencies in his argument for value-free science and the separation of the scientific from the political role. The difficulty with this solution, however, is that (a) value inputs penetrate deeply behind the wall of the scientific stage and (b) that virtually all scientific activity has at least some application component. This leads us to a third model for the application stage.

c. *The Collegial Model*. Our third model for the application stage arises from the criticism of the first two. The technical expert in the collegial model is granted no peculiar expertise in evaluation; there is no generalization of expertise. On the other hand he must accept moral responsibility for the reasonably foreseeable implications of his research and advice. If the layman in the technological action system is treated as a colleague his values are to be taken into account as well as the technical expert's.[58] The technical expert should place heavy emphasis upon maximizing the layman's value inputs into decision-making so that the process becomes a corporate effort. At the same time it must be realistically admitted that value inputs penetrate so deeply into the scientific stage that the technical expert is never acting in a value-free manner. This is neither possible nor morally acceptable.

The difficulty with the collegial model is that it requires collegiality. It can only be appropriate when the substructural factors in the technical expert-layman relationship do, in fact, reflect collegial status. There must be some common ground in status, authority, economic position, as well as world view. Unfortunately this is only rarely the case in professional-lay relationships today. It is dangerous and paternalistic to pretend collegiality.

d. *The Contractual Model.* There is still a fourth alternative, one which retains the balance of professional and lay value inputs. For this reason we might call both the collegial and contractual models "balanced." The contractual model differs, however, from the collegial model in that it does not require the degree of substructural harmony and personalistic relationship necessary for the interaction among colleagues.

In Chapter II we argued that the interaction between the professional and lay actors was not undirectional. There is an instrumental contribution by the professional which is often seen as the major element, but there is also an instrumental contribution by the lay actor. Likewise there are expressive (cathectic and evaluative) contributions by both. These exchanges can be conceptualized as elements of a contractual relation. If they are seen as parts of a contract in which both professional and layman have instrumental and expressive rights and obligations within a limited context, the abuses of the clinical and engineering models can be avoided. It also can avoid the artificiality of the collegial model.

Gerard Egan, in a paper called "Contractual Approaches to the Control and Modification of Behavior in Encounter Groups," has suggested that the contractual model is the most appropriate for the relationship between professional and layman in the field of psychology.[59] It is the one relationship which permits both the freedom and responsibility necessary for decision-making in which the professional has clear expertise in one area (the technical data), but only limited authority in other areas (the evaluative).

While the contractual model is familiar to Western secular society, it also has religious, theological roots in the

Judeo-Christian tradition. In its secular form the contract permits the restriction and protection necessary for both parties in the relationship. In its religious form the covenant permits the development of respect, trust, and faith which are essential for the professional-lay relationship. Only by developing the image of the contract-covenant, either implicitly or explicitly, will the abuses of evaluation inherent in the clinical, engineering, and collegial models of the scientific and technological decision-making process be overcome.

This completes our analysis of the value factors in the scientific and technological process--the pre-scientific, scientific, and post-scientific stages--and also brings to a close the theoretical formulations which constitute the first part of this volume. In Part II we shall attempt to illustrate the themes which have been developed thus far by examining in detail a specific example of the scientific and technological decision-making process--the physician's decisions regarding oral contraceptives.

[1]For the discussions of the theory of decision-making, see Nicholas Rescher, *Introduction to Value Theory* (Englewood Cliffs, N.J.: Prentice-Hall, Inc., 1969), pp. 29-48; James Bates, "A Model for the Science of Decision," *Philosophy of Science*, XXI (1954), pp. 326-39; Donald Davidson, Patrick Suppes, and Sidney Siegel, *Decision-Making: An Experimental Approach* (Stanford: Stanford University Press, 1957); Nicholas M. Smith, Jr., Stanley S. Walters, Franklin C. Brooks, and David H. Blackwell, "The Theory of Value and the Science of Decision: A Summary," *Journal of the Operations Research Society of America*, I (1953), pp. 103-13; and Arnold Kaufman, *The Science of Decision-Making* (London: Weidenfeld, 1968).

[2]In this simplified model we appear to be suggesting that values are utterly distinct from facts. We have not said this, however. In fact we do not hold that to be the case at all. We shall discuss this below.

[3]See Richard B. Brandt, *Ethical Theory: The Problems of Normative and Critical Ethics*, (Englewood Cliffs, N.J.: Prentice-Hall, Inc., 1959), p. 231-39.

[4]See Stephen Grant Young, "Parent and Child - Compulsory Medical Care Over Objections of Parents," *West Virginia Law Review*, LXV (1963), pp. 184-87.

[5]A recent example of value-loaded fact is the publication of a study on the level of unwanted fertility in the United States. The authors claim (presumably on sound basis) that seventeen percent of all children of parents in the study are unwanted at time of birth. They suggest that, assuming no reduction in subfecundity, prevention of these births would eliminate a major portion of our growth rate. They make no policy claims in the article, but this article is now appearing very frequently as scientific evidence for the correctness of a voluntary family planning policy for this country. Their work has taken on the status of value-loaded fact.
Working from their data a different set of value-loaded facts could also be stated: (a) Even under the above assumptions approximately one-third of the growth rate would remain. (b) It is very unlikely that a contraceptive method which is ethically and medically universally acceptable will be developed in the foreseeable future. (c) There are likely to be breakthroughs permitting the reduction of subfecundity. (d) The resulting rate of growth would be projected to be almost identical with the present actual growth in this group. These statements are entirely consistent with the one made above. These are value-loaded facts opposing a voluntary population policy. It should be clear that neither of these presumably reliable sets of statements of fact is sufficient in itself for determination of a policy decision.

Larry Bumpass and Charles F. Westoff, "The Perfect Contraceptive-Population," *Science* (Sept. 18, 1970), pp. 1177-82, is the main published account of the number of unwanted births in the United States. For some countervailing value-loaded observations, see Judith Blake, "Reproductive Motivation and Population Policy," *BioScience* (March 1, 1971), p. 217.

[6]John Locke, *Essay Concerning Human Understanding*, in *Locke Selections*, ed. by Sterling P. Lamprecht (New York: Charles Scribner's Sons, 1928), p. 207.

[7]Francis Hutcheson, *Introduction to Moral Philosophy in Three Books Containing the Elements of Ethics and Law of Nature* (Glasgow: Robert and Andrew Foulis, 1753), p. 16.

[8]G. E. Moore, *Principia Ethica* (Cambridge, England: Cambridge University Press, 1966), p. 7.

[9]*Ibid*

[10]*Ibid.*, p. 13.

[11]W. K. Frankena, "The Naturalistic Fallacy," in *Readings in Ethical Theory*, ed. by Wilfred Sellars and John Hospers (New York: Appleton-Century-Crofts, Inc., 1952), pp. 103-14.

[12]*Ibid.*, p. 109.

[13]See Stephen C. Pepper, "A Brief History of General Theory of Value," in *A History of Philosophical Systems*, ed. by V. Ferm (New York, 1950), pp. 500-01.

[14]Roderick Firth, "Ethical Absolutism and the Ideal Observer," *Philosophy and Phenomenological Research*, XII, No. 3 (March, 1952), pp. 317-45.

[15]Arthur J. Dyck, "A Gestalt Analysis of the Moral Data and Certain of its Implications for Ethical Theory," (unpublished Ph.D. dissertation, Harvard University, 1965).

[16]Firth, p. 323.

[17]*Ibid.*, p. 324.

[18]Firth, in a personal communication with this author, accepted this slight reformulation of his analysis which stresses the properties in the ethical phenomena themselves.

[19]Read Bain, "Science, Values, and Sociology," *American Sociological Review*, IV (August, 1937), 562.

[20]Max Weber, "Objectivity in Social Science and Social Policy," in *The Methodology of the Social Science* (New York: The Free Press, 1949), p. 21.

[21]Talcott Parsons, "Evaluation and Objectivity in Social Science," in *Sociological Theory and Modern Society* (New York: The Free Press, 1967), p. 86-87.

[22]Aristotle, *The Nichomachean Ethics*, I, 7, ed. by Martin Oswald (Indianapolis: Bobbs-Merrill, 1962), p. 15.

[23]W. D. Ross, *The Right and the Good* (Oxford: Oxford University Press, 1930), p. 140.

[24]Wolfgang Köhler, *The Place of Value in the World of Facts* (New York: New American Library, 1966), p. 39.

[25]See Ralf Dahrendorf, "Values and Social Science," in *Essay in the Theory of Society* (Stanford: Stanford University Press, 1968), p. 7.

[26]The actual studies have not been published. Accounts on the debate have been reported in "A Diabetes Tea Party Hits FDA," *Medical World News* (Dec. 18, 1970), pp. 13-14, and "The Tolbutamide Debate," *Medical World News* (Jan. 8, 1970), pp. 37-46.

[27]"A Diabetes Tea Party," p. 13.

[28]Weber, "Objectivity," p. 60.

[29]Max Weber, "The Meaning of 'Ethical Neutrality' in Sociology and Economics," in *The Methodology of the Social Sciences* (New York: The Free Press, 1949), p. 11.

[30]*Ibid.*

[31]Dahrendorf, "Values and Social Science," p. 11.

[32]Herbert Marcuse, *One-Dimensional Man* (Boston: Beacon Press, 1964), p. 19.

[33]Theodore J. Gordon, "The Feedback Between Technology and Values," in *Values and the Future*, ed. by Kurt Baier and Nicholas Rescher (New York: The Free Press, 1969), pp. 148-92. Also see Robert Boguslaw, *The New Utopians* (Englewood Cliffs, N.J.: Prentice-Hall, Inc., 1968), p. 23.

[34]See Robert Rosenthal and Lenore Jacobson, *Pygmalian in the Classroom* (New York: Holt, Rinehart, and Winston, 1968).

[35]Robert Rosenthal, *Experimenter Effects in Behavioural Research* (New York: Appleton Crofts, 1966).

[36]Dahrendorf, "Values and Social Science," p. 10.

[37]Weber makes this separation explicit in "The Logic of the Cultural Sciences," in *The Methodology of the Social Sciences* (New York: The Free Press, 1949), p. 176.

[38]Boguslaw, *The New Utopians*.

[39]Robert K. Merton, "The Bearing of Empirical Research on Sociological Theory," in *On Theoretical Sociology* (New York: The Free Press, 1967), pp. 156-71.

[40]G. Burch, "The Use of the Proper Theoretical Models in the Scientific Study of Religion," (unpublished paper, 1970).

[41]Robert W. Friedrichs, *A Sociology of Sociology* (New York: The Free Press, 1970).

[42]Han Young Kim, "Balance and Dissonance Theories of the Adoption and Diffusion of an Innovation Applied to the IUCD," *Social Biology*, XVII, No. 1 (March, 1970), pp. 43-53.

[43]John Walton, "Discipline, Method, and Community Power: A Note on the Sociology of Knowledge," *American Sociological Review*, XXXI (1966), pp. 684-89.

[44]Jane Cassels Record, "The Research Institute and the Pressure Group," in *Ethics, Politics, and Social Research*, ed. by Gideon Sjoberg (Cambridge, Mass.: Schenkman Publishing Co., Inc., 1967), p. 40.

[45]Pierre L. van den Berghe, "Research in South Africa: The Story of My Experiences with Tyranny," in *ibid.*, p. 189.

[46]T. N. Madan, "Political Pressures and Ethical Constraints Upon Indian Sociologists," in *ibid.*, p. 171.

[47]See Leonard D. Cain, Jr., "The AMA and the Gerontologists: Uses and Abuses of 'A Profile of the Aging: USA,'" in *ibid.*, pp. 78-114, for a striking example of the significance of sample selection.

[48]Richard A. Brymer and Buford Farris, "Ethical and Political Dilemmas in the Investigation of Deviance: A Study of Juvenile Delinquency," in *ibid.*, p. 315. Also see Richard Colvard, "Interaction and Identification in Reporting Field Research: A Critical Reconsideration of Protective Procedures," *ibid.*, p. 319 (italics added).

[49]Herbert C. Kelman, *A Time to Speak: On Human Values and Social Research* (San Francisco: Jossey-Bass, Inc., 1968).

[50]See "Privacy and Behavioral Research," (Washington, D.C.: Executive Office of the President, Office of Science and Technology, 1967); "Ethical Aspects of Experimentation with Human Subjects," *Daedalus* (Spring, 1969); and Herbert C. Kelman, "The Human Use of Human Subjects," in *A Time to Speak*, pp. 208-25, for some of this discussion.

[51]Ted R. Vaughan, "Governmental Intervention in Social Research: Political and Ethical Dimensions in the Wichita Jury Recordings," in *Ethics, Politics, and Social Research*, p. 71.

[52]Kelman, *A Time to Speak*, pp. 8-105.

[53]Ernst Troeltsch, "Das stoisch-christliche Naturrecht und die moderne profane Naturrecht," *Gesammelte Schriften*, IV (Tübingen: Verlag J. C. B. Mohr [Paul Siebeck], 1925), pp. 166-91.

[54]Robert Boguslaw, "Values in the Research Society," in *The Research Society*, ed. by E. Glatt and M. W. Shelley (New York: Gordon and Breach, 1968), p. 53, makes the point saying that "Large scale research activities demand funds. And funds disbursed by foundations, governments, or even philanthropists are not ordinarily available in large quantities to satisfy the idle, recreational interests of other people, even if these other people call themselves scientists."

[55]Robert N. Wilson, *The Sociology of Health: An Introduction* (New York: Random House, 1970), pp. 18, 20.

[56]Weber, "The Meaning of 'Ethical Neutrality'," p. 4.

[57]For discussion of Project Camelot, see Irving Louis Horowitz, ed., *The Rise and Fall of Project Camelot* (Cambridge, Mass.: The M.I.T. Press, 1967); also Kelman, *A Time to Speak*, pp. 59ff, 92ff.

[58]For an example of the development of the collegial model for the experimenter-subject relationship, see Talcott Parsons, "Research with Human Subjects and the 'Professional Complex'," in *Daedalus* (Spring, 1969), pp. 325-60.

[59]Gerard Egan, "Contractual Approaches to the Control and Modification of Behavior in Encounter Groups" (unpublished paper presented at the 1970 meetings of the American Association for the Advancement of Science).

PART II

A CASE STUDY OF MEDICAL DECISIONS

ON CONTRACEPTION

CHAPTER V

BIRTH CONTROL AND THE PHYSICIAN: WHAT IS KNOWN

In Part I we have presented a theoretical framework for consideration of the relation between scientific and technological decision-making and religious, ethical, and other sociocultural factors. Now we shall examine a specific area of decision-making in order to illustrate some of the themes developed in the theoretical discussion.

The area we have chosen is physician decision-making regarding oral contraception. First, in Chapter V, we shall review what is known about the attitudes and practices of physicians related to contraception. In Chapter VI we shall attempt to develop the dimensions of the cultural value complex related to oral contraception by examining statements of relevant groups. In Chapter VII we shall present the results of an empirical study of physicians' values and their decision-making on oral contraception. Finally in the last chapter we shall discuss in a more detailed way the relationship of the physician's views to those of his patients based upon a more thorough study of one particular community.

INTRODUCTION

In a 1957 study, one-third of all Catholic obstetricians and gynecologists believed rhythm to be "the most *reliable* contraceptive procedure." Of even more interest, two percent of all non-Catholic physicians in the study held this view.[1] Of all Catholic physicians who claim to decide about contraception mainly on medical rather than moral grounds, two-fifths disapproved of appliance methods.[2]

Since all medical scientists in the United States have at their disposal virtually the same scientific information, a naive view of scientific rational medicine would suggest that physicians should agree about general principles of efficaciousness and safety. Obviously this is not the case. Within the broad limits set by technical information, medical decision-making is greatly influenced by psychological, social, and

cultural factors. In the area of family planning these factors
are very pronounced. In this chapter we shall review the small
body of literature available on the influence of social and
cultural factors on these decisions. Then in Chapter VII we
shall present some preliminary research of our own in the area.

When one realizes that for the four most effective means
of controlling births[3] and for one of the two next most effective methods the physician's approval for use is required by
law, it is surprising that almost no attention has been given
to the holders of this contraceptive veto power.[4]

We would particularly like to know what happens when a
physician and patient have differences in these social and cultural factors. Spivack found that among the physicians he
studied, forty-five percent of the patients of Catholics were
non-Catholic. Among non-Catholics thirty-two percent of the
patients were Catholic.[5] We also are interested in the extent
to which social and cultural factors influence presumably scientific readings of (non-evaluative) facts.

In a debate occurring in a medical journal, a Dr. Cunningham argues:

> The action of the pill then seems to be, in
> a proportion of cases, abortion of the fertilized
> ovum. I am concerned about this destruction of
> human life from a moral standpoint and also from
> a public health standpoint. Delayed imbedding of
> a fertilized ovum may lead to a deformed or
> retarded child.[6]

In a reply in the same journal, Dr. Gordon W. Perkin offered a theological argument quoting the British Council of
Churches to the effect that even if the fertilized egg is de-
stroyed before nidation there is no moral offense. Then he
concludes:

> A survey of all the medical literature pub-
> lished on the use of the present oral contracep-
> tives reveals no evidence to suggest such a
> possible relationship [between oral contraceptives
> and deformed children].[7]

The interaction of each moral-theological argument with
the corresponding opinions about action on the fertilized ovum
and deformed children seems likely. We shall not take up in

detail in this discussion the related question of how important
the physician is as a source of birth control information as
compared with other sources. Spivack's study revealed that
only twenty-seven percent of physicians considered themselves
the primary source of women's information on birth control.[8]
Bakker and Dightman's study of women's information gave a figure
of thirty-seven percent.[9] In our own studies we found that one
quarter of seventy-nine unmarried students at a Catholic girls
college gave a physician as one of their two most important
sources of information.

There appears to be a connection between physicians' lack
of willingness to take the initiative in birth control discussion and their low ranking as a source of information which in
turn has been connected to their cultural attitudes and their
lack of training in the area in medical schools.[10] Spivack's
study in 1957 revealed that forty-seven percent of physicians
"never" take the initiative in discussing contraception in the
premarital examination. Fifty percent "hardly ever" or "never"
take the initiative in the postpartum examination.[11] There appears to have been substantial change in physician willingness
to initiate conversations over the past few years. In an unpublished study of physicians in two counties in California in
1965, Barnes *et al.* found that fifty-nine percent said that
they should initiate family planning conversations with their
patients.[12] In our own study discussed in Chapter VII, we
shall present more comparable data showing even more movement
toward initiation of conversations by physicians. This apparent change in decision-making seems to be a reflection of the
feedback loop in which the existence of a new technology has an
impact on values. This feedback was discussed in Chapter IV.
Several authors support Nash's postulation that:

> patients would prefer the physician to take more
> initiative in relation to discussion of the var-
> ious methods of contraception, especially at times
> when he might consider it possible that another
> pregnancy would be unwise for any reason.[13]

but firm studies to establish this point are lacking.

Before beginning our review of how cultural and social
factors affect physicians' family planning attitudes we shall

summarize in table form the studies from which our information
has been drawn.

Spengler's model for analysis of fertility includes three
factors: total income, relative costs of fertility behavior
patterns as determined by the price system, and the preference
system.[14] He is particularly interested in pursuing study of
the preference system and its relationship to goals and values.
The literature frequently minimizes the significance of values
in fertility analysis due to their presumed stability.[15]

While Spengler's model was intended for analysis of
couple's fertility behavior, it is also useful for study of the
behavior of other social units such as a legislature or in our
case a physician. Here a balance of competing value systems
may be operating in a delicate balance. Particularly where a
patient's freedom of choice of physician is emphasized, shifts
in behavior can be brought about with only minor shifts in a
preference system. One need not change value commitments of a
patient other than those expressed in choice of a physician.

In any case, it becomes important to know how the physician's value choices and socio-cultural frame of reference are
expressed in his practice, and we shall move now to a review of
these factors.

A. RELIGION

Spivack's major study concluded that:

> While specialty, age of doctor, professional
> status, and community factors account for much
> variation among doctors in one or another as-
> pect of family-planning behavior, the religion
> of the doctor is even more influential.[16]

> The basic disagreement among doctors is on the
> means for achieving family planning, and this
> disagreement is based not on medical but pri-
> marily on religious grounds.[17]

In spite of this seemingly reasonable conclusion, only the
Spivack study among those studies of physicians listed in Table
1 which deal with contraception includes religion as an important variable.[18] This would appear to be a serious flaw in
experimental design in the studies we are considering.

TABLE 1

EMPIRICAL STUDIES OF PHYSICIANS' ATTITUDES AND PRACTICES

Year of Study	Senior Researcher	Sample Size	Sample Characteristics
1944	Guttmacher[1]	3381	National random sample plus all ob-gyn
1957	Spivack[2]	551	6 communities; high and low Catholic pairs for city, town, and rural
1950-60	Hall[3]	60 hospitals	[primarily on abortion]
[published 1964]	Herndon and Nash[4]	514	22% random sample Medical Society of North Carolina (whites only)
[published 1964]	Lief[5]	20	Tulane University Teaching Staff
[published 1964]	Medical Tribune[6]	1300	National [on abortion]
1964	Eliot[7] (Committee on Family and Population Planning of the Maternal and Child Health Section, A.P.H.A.)	40	Chief of obstetrics and one resident at 20 hospitals (5 Catholic) in one metropolitan area
1964	Landis[8]	770	Active members of the county medical society in Northern California [on vasectomy]
1964	Tietze[9]	94 Medical Schools	78 Non-Catholic U.S. 7 Catholic U.S. 9 Canada
1964	Siegel[10]	20 clinicians 9 public health officers 181 public health nurses	15% stratified random sample of health departments of California plus randomly selected sample of clinicians
[published 1964]	Medical Tribune[11]	1159	poll respondents

TABLE 1--continued

Year of Study	Senior Researcher	Sample Size	Sample Characteristics
[published 1965]	Bakker[12]	109 physicians 100 "women" (not physicians)	53 ob-gyn 56 general practitioners
1965	Barnes[13]	188	California physicians
1965	Hall[14]	1350	New York ob-gyn [on abortion]
1965	Wright[15]	212	Georgia county public health clinic physicians
[published 1966]	Sherwin[16]	748	California ob-gyn [on abortion]
1966	Crowley[17]	5289	American Psychiatric Association members [on abortion]
[published 1967]	Lyle[18]	6733	National, members of the American College of Obstetrics and Gynecology
1967	Eliot[19]	372	Hospital chiefs of obstetrics [on abortion]
1968	Eliot[20]	about 3000	Michigan physicians [on abortion]
1969	Modern Medicine[21]	27,741	[on abortion]
[published 1969]	Wolf[22]	"over 300 patients"	inner city Baltimore patients
[published 1970]	Smith[23]	425	Hawaiian Medical Association [on abortion]

[1]Alan F. Guttmacher, "Conception Control and the Medical Profession," *Human Fertility*, XII, No. 1 (March, 1947), pp. 1-10.

[2]Sydney S. Spivack, "Religious Attitudes of Physicians and Dissemination of Contraceptive Advice," (unpublished Ph.D. dissertation, Columbia University, 1959); Sydney S. Spivack, "The

Doctor's Role in Family Planning," *Journal of the American Medical Association*, CLXXXVIII, No. 2 (April 13, 1964), pp. 152-56; Sydney S. Spivack, "Family Planning in Medical Practice," in *Research in Family Planning*, ed. by Clyde V. Kiser (Princeton: Princeton University Press, 1962), pp. 193-210; and Mary Jean Cornish, Florence Ruderman, and Sydney S. Spivack, *Doctors and Family Planning* (New York: National Committee on Maternal Health, Inc., 1963).

[3]Robert E. Hall, "Therapeutic Abortion, Sterilization and Contraception," *American Journal of Obstetrics and Gynecology*, XCI (1965), pp. 518-32.

[4]E. M. Nash, "Attitudes of Physicians Affecting Contraceptive Practice, in Mary S. Calderone, ed., *Manual of Contraceptive Practice* (Baltimore: Williams and Wilkins, 1964), pp. 96-103; and C. N. Herndon and E. M. Nash, "Premarriage and Marriage Counselling: A Study of Practices of North Carolina Physicians," *Journal of the American Medical Association* LXXX (1962), pp. 395-99.

[5]H. I. Lief, "Sexual Attitudes and Behavior of Medical Students: Implications for Medical Practice," in E. M. Nash, *et al.*, *Marriage Counseling in Medical Practice* (Chapel Hill, N.C.: University of North Carolina Press, 1964), pp. 301-08.

[6]"Social, Economic Basis for Abortion Upheld," *Medical Tribune* (October 31-November 1, 1964), pp. 21-22.

[7]Johan W. Eliot and Gitta Meier, "Fertility Control in Hospitals with Residencies in Obstetrics and Gynecology," *Obstetrics and Gynecology*, XXVIII (October, 1966), pp. 582-91.

[8]Judson Landis, "Attitudes of Individual California Physicians and Policies of State Medical Societies on Vasectomy for Birth Control," *Journal of Marriage and the Family*, XXVIII, No. 3 (August, 1966), pp. 277-83.

[9]Christopher Tietze, *et al.*, "Teaching of Fertility Regulation in Medical Schools: Survey of United States and Canada, 1964," *Journal of the American Medical Association*, XCCVI, No. 1 (April 4, 1966), pp. 20-24.

[10]Earl Siegel and Ronald C. Dillehay, "Some Approaches to Family Planning Counseling in Local Health Departments: A Survey of Public Health Nurses and Physicians," *American Journal of Public Health*, LVI (November, 1966), pp. 1840-46.

[11]"Most M.D.'s Favor Birth Control Data for Patients," *Medical Tribune* (May 23-24, 1964), pp. 15 and 21.

[12]Cornelius C. Bakker and Cameron R. Dightman, "Physicians and Family Planning: A Persistent Ambivalence," *Obstetrics and Gynecology*, XXV (February, 1965), pp. 279-84.

[13]John Barnes, Larry Johnson, Helen Kaufman, William Nichols, and Peter Olsson, "Attitudes and Practices of Physicians Concerning Birth Control in Two California Counties," 1965 (unpublished manuscript).

[14]Robert Hall, "New York Abortion Law Survey," *American Journal of Obstetrics and Gynecology*, XCIII, No. 8 (December 15, 1965), pp. 1182-83.

[15]Nicholas M. Wright, George Johnson, and Donald Mees, "Georgia Physicians' Attitudes Toward Family Planning Services, Prescribing Contraceptives, Sex Education, and Therapeutic Abortion: Report of a Survey" (unpublished manuscript, no date [1966?]).

[16]Lawrence Sherwin and Edmund W. Overstreet, "Therapeutic Abortion: Attitudes and Practices of California Physicians," *California Medicine*, CV (November, 1966), pp. 337-39.

[17]Ralph M. Crowley and Robert W. Laidlaw, "Psychiatric Opinion Regarding Abortion: Preliminary Report of a Survey," *American Journal of Psychiatry*, CXXIV, No. 4 (October, 1967), pp. 145-48.

[18]Alice Lake, "The Pill," *McCalls* (November, 1967), pp. 96-97 and *passim*.

[19]Johan W. Eliot, Robert E. Hall, J. Robert Wilson, and Carolyn Houser, "The Obstetrician's View," in *Abortion in a Changing World*, I, ed. by Robert E. Hall (New York: Columbia University Press, 1970), pp. 85-95.

[20]Johan W. Eliot, Jack Stack, Roy Smith, and Patricia Sullivan, "Michigan Physicians' Views on Changing Michigan Abortion Laws and Experience with Abortion Requests." (Unpublished manuscript.)

[21]"Modern Medicine Poll on Sociomedical Issues: Abortion--Homosexual Practices--Marihuana," *Modern Medicine* (November 3, 1969), pp. 18-25.

[22]Sanford R. Wolf and Elsie L. Ferguson, "The Physician's Influence on the Nonacceptance of Birth Control," *American Journal of Obstetrics and Gynecology*, CIV, No. 5 (July 1, 1969), pp. 752-57.

[23]Roy G. Smith, "Changing Hawaii's Abortion Laws," *Public Health*, III (1970), pp. 2-4.

1. *When Religion Is Expressed.*

The position of the Catholic Church, though often misunderstood in detail, is well known in principle. A text on Catholic medical ethics states:

> no instruction on the methods of using contraceptives of any type may be given to any person, regardless of religion....No advice or encouragement to use contraceptives may be given to any person....[19]

This position is reflected in actual practice, but not in as simple a way as most believe. A non-Catholic doctor is seven times as likely to consider providing contraceptive advice and information a "standard procedure" than is a Catholic (twenty-nine percent to four percent).[20] Fifty-nine percent of the Catholic general practitioners, internists, and obstetricians in Spivack's study believe "no advice should be given" or "advice about rhythm only should be given"[21] (cf. one percent of non-Catholics). The following table, based on Spivack's data, indicates differences based on religion are not limited to practices related to banned contraceptive devices, but extend to a broad area of marital and family planning counseling:

TABLE 2

DIFFERENCES IN PRACTICES OF CATHOLICS AND NON-CATHOLICS, 1957[22]

	Non-Catholic	Catholic
Provide marital counseling frequently	48%	37%
Introduce subject of contraception often or very frequently in premarital exam	40%	10%
Introduce subject of child spacing sometimes or almost always with postpartum patients	59%	20%
Practice includes fitting diaphragm	24%	14%

Disapproval of chemical or mechanical contraception among Catholic doctors was found to be associated with frequent church attendance, considering religion important, attending a

Catholic medical school, being affiliated with a Catholic hospital, and having Catholic colleagues.[23]

In two California counties Barnes *et al.* found that in 1965 fifty-five percent of the Catholic general practitioners, internists, and obstetrician-gynecologists approved of chemical or mechanical methods of birth control compared with 99.4% of the non-Catholics.[24] Fifty percent of the Catholics would provide birth control counselling or service to childless, unmarried women compared with eighty-five percent of the non-Catholics.[25]

In terms of our theoretical formulation in Chapter II, religious affiliation is a major variable coming from the sphere of the actor's social system (see Figures 3 and 4). We are not dealing directly with the symbol system which is the direct locus of the decision-making process. To the extent that religious affiliation enters that decision-making process at all, it does so through what we called the secondary factor of cathectic or expressive symbolization (Figure 7). Religious affiliation may have great impact on the formulation of the evaluative system which is a primary factor (the major premise as we have discussed it in Chapter IV) of the decision-making process. It is an oversimplification brought about by a sociological bias facilitated by ease of measure which has led social scientists to focus upon religious affiliation rather than the system of evaluation as a major variable in studying birth control.

2. *When Religion Is Not Religion: Disguised Expressions of Cultural Values.*

While differences in practice are to be expected, differences in presumably scientific and technical decisions are also quite apparent. We have noted that one in three Catholic obstetricians in the Spivack study believed rhythm to be the most reliable means of contraception. In a hypothetical case of a severe cardiac patient who requested to be taught rhythm only twenty percent of Catholic doctors would urge other methods compared to sixty-six percent of the non-Catholics. Many Catholics commented that "because of advances in medicine a cardiac condition does not typically contraindicate pregnancy."[26]

Thirty-five percent of Catholics believe judgments should be based primarily on medical grounds (cf. 80% of non-Catholics). Of these we have noted that two in five still disapprove of appliance methods. The interaction of cultural values and scientific judgments seems apparent in these cases, but until now there has been no systematic study of these relations. The recognition of expression of a cultural value through scientific claims (which are more acceptable in presumably rational Western medicine) may be critically important because it is so disguised. Our own study to be described in Chapter VII attempts to measure specifically just this interaction.

In terms of the model of the scientific action system developed in Chapter II there is an interaction between the (non-evaluative) cognitive symbolization and the evaluative symbolization in the cultural system. This gives rise to value inputs into the handling of information at the descriptive, scientific stage giving rise either to biasing and distortion of information (Type IIC) or selection of the information considered "relevant" (Type IID). Through these phenomena so-called facts become what we have called "value-loaded."

3. *When Cultural Values Are Not Institutional Religion.*

The recent national study of the American College of Obstetrics and Gynecology reports that only four percent of all obstetricians said that religious considerations prevented them from prescribing the "pill."[27] This appears to reduce religion to a trivial consideration. The problem, however, is much more complex. We have already reported data suggesting there is considerable "spill over" of cultural level values into "scientific" decisions. The great differences in behavior between Catholic and non-Catholic doctors in spite of the fact that most might prescribe the "pill" at least on occasion indicate an important variable.

An even greater problem is that even when a cultural value complex is considered, which we have argued has a religious component, the stereotype of Catholic vs. non-Catholic breaks

down. What is really significant is a large but vague cultural
value complex which is related only imperfectly to religious
affiliation. Many non-Catholics have very "Catholic" attitudes
toward family planning and vice versa. Thus in one of the fifteen non-Catholic obstetrics residency programs studied by
Eliot, there was no instruction in family planning, their
clinic had no family planning service and both the chief of
staff and the resident saw no place for family planning in the
hospital program.[28] On the other hand, many Catholics are en-
thusiastic about all forms of birth control. To our knowledge
no study has attempted to measure this broad value complex and
use it as a variable rather than the overly simple religious
affiliation indicator. This is one of the objectives of the
work we shall describe below.

4. *When the Patient and Physician Have Different Cultural
    Values.*

What happens in the case of interaction of conflicting
value systems is almost completely unknown. Catholic Church
policy is that physicians may teach only rhythm and may not refer patients to non-Catholic physicians even if the patient is
not Catholic.[29] This directly opposes the AMA position that it
is the responsibility of conscientiously objecting physicians
to "refer the patients to appropriate persons."[30]

It is known that physicians dealing with patients of a
different religion tend to treat them according to the physician's value system. In 1957 a non-Catholic had one chance in
four of getting a contraceptive device prescribed from a Catholic doctor.[31]

A very critical question is what happens to a patient who
is refused service by a physician or hospital. How much initiative is taken in going to another source? What percentage
of refusals are on presumably medical grounds and what is the
effect of this on seeking further advice? How significant is
the effect of lack of physician initiative? Research into
these questions could probably best be undertaken in national
fertility studies rather than through studies of physicians.
The demographic consequences of the cultural components in the
patient-physician interaction are as yet unstudied.

B. MEDICAL EDUCATION

While religious or cultural values are probably the most important variable in physician attitudes and practices, other socio-cultural variables also come into play. Probably next in importance is the institutional influence of the physician's medical education.

Tietze's study of medical schools in 1964 revealed twelve non-Catholic schools where rhythm was taught as a "preferred" method. Two others considered aerosol "preferred."[32] This study, done for the American Public Health Association, reveals an important source of physicians' diverging opinions as well as documenting the often reported charge that "doctors are woefully ignorant about sex"[33] or at least seriously deficient in training in family planning.[34] In 1944, 74.9% of physicians indicated they had no training in contraception.[35] By 1964, while seventy-one of seventy-eight non-Catholic schools included contraception in the regular curriculum, half had less than two hours in the four year program. Less than half examined their students on the subject. In seven Catholic schools only one teaches methods other than rhythm. Only one school has a formal lecture on the subject, one hour in four years. Only thirteen of thirty-eight obstetrics-gynecology texts written in the last ten years have more than passing mention of contraception and even here there is gross disagreement.[36]

There have been no attempts to relate physicians' practices to their schools or to determine the adequacy of postgraduate training. Much could be done with already gathered data. Several studies have asked for schools attended. Nevertheless, all of this information takes into account only the crude sociological variable of religious affiliation of the medical school. We would argue that only when the ethical and other values in the system of evaluation of the policy makers at the medical school are considered more directly and together with the formal and informal transferring of this evaluative system in the process of socialization of the student will it be possible to have any real understanding of the importance of medical education in shaping the patterns of thought and behavior of the physician.

C. TYPES OF MEDICAL PRACTICE

Eliot's study of hospital residencies in obstetrics and related family planning clinics provides the best information in areas other than private practice.[37] There are no studies comparing types of practice (solo, group, prepaid health corporations, etc.). In general, Eliot's findings were similar to Tietze's study of schools. Most residencies give little or no training in family planning, but there are great differences among hospitals. Although most of the non-Catholic hospitals had no hospital-wide policies covering family planning, Eliot concluded that absence of restrictive policy was not enough to insure adequate services.[38] This illustrates the importance of looking beyond religious affiliation. Individual initiative varied considerably. Particularly critical was the active interest of the chief of staff. This in turn we would suggest is related to the cultural values complex, but there are no data on the subject. One Catholic and one non-Catholic hospital (out of a total of twenty) had no instruction and no service in family planning and considered it unessential.

Hall's study of sixty hospitals revealed a 3.6 times higher rate of therapeutic abortions in private services than in wards.[39] He suggests that similar biases exist with regard to contraceptive advice, but admits there is no firm evidence. Twenty-two of thirty-seven hospitals reporting indicated contraceptive advice was available to less than twenty-six percent of their patients.[40] (Thirteen offered it to none.) He suggests higher percentages for private patients. Further work in the area would prove interesting. Either physician surveys or participant-observer reporting in a hospital setting could be used. In Chapter VIII we shall report an in-depth study of one hospital's obstetrics staff.

Siegel's recent study of California Boards of Health is the only research into the public health field. He compared public health nurses with physicians, but his physician sample included twenty in private practice and eight maternal and child health administrators, making the results of less value for our purposes.[41] He found 35.7% of his physicians would initiate family planning discussion compared to 53.8% of the public health nurses.[42]

Eliot's study of Michigan physicians' attitudes on abortion is interesting because it is the only one to our knowledge which included osteopathic physicians in its sample. They appear to have similar views on abortion to their non-osteopathic counterparts. Eighty-four percent of the 558 osteopathic physicians surveyed favored elimination or replacement of the Michigan law while eighty-seven percent of the medical physicians took the same position.[43]

Virtually nothing is known about the effect of politics on the financing of publicly supported services, although several hospital administrators indicated they were cautious about including family planning budget items for fear of political and monetary consequences.[44]

D. OTHER SOCIOLOGICAL VARIABLES

Typical background data categories for sociological analysis have been analyzed only tangentially and then only in a few studies, particularly Guttmacher's and Spivack's.

1. *Age*.

Bakker and Dightman[45] found year of graduation to be insignificant in predicting attitudes and practices. Eliot, in his study of Michigan physicians' attitudes on abortion, divided his respondents into groups by age. For groups below thirty, thirty to thirty-nine, forty to forty-nine, and fifty and up, he found little difference in opinion about whether they wanted the present law either eliminated or revised. For all the groups from 86.3 to 88.5 percent wanted either elimination or revision.[46] The study of Barnes *et al.* analyzed data by comparing those who had been in practice less than ten years with those in practice more than twenty-five years. They found a consistent pattern of the physicians who had been in practice a shorter period being more inclined to "advise about birth control even though advice is not sought," to "prescribe to unmarried patients who seek the advice," to prescribe the IUD or the pill rather than the diaphragm, and to provide birth control counselling or services to unmarried women. The differences, however, were small; eighty-one percent of physicians

in practice under ten years compared with seventy-four percent
of physicians in practice over twenty-five years would provide
birth control counselling or services to childless unmarried
women.[47]

Nevertheless, several studies indicate that next to religion, age is the most critical variable. A *Modern Medicine*
poll asking "Should abortion be available to any woman capable
of giving legal consent upon her own request to a competent
physician?" was affirmed without qualification by fifty-seven
percent of the physicians responding who were under thirty-five
but by only forty-four percent of those over sixty-five.[48] Using year of graduation as an indicator, Guttmacher, in 1941,
found that of those who graduated before 1910, 57.4% preferred
diaphragms. Of those graduating after 1935, 83.7% did.[49]
Spivack, in 1957, found that for non-Catholic doctors under
thirty-five, fifty percent considered providing contraceptive
advice a "standard procedure," while only fifteen percent of
those over sixty-five did.[50] Nevertheless he found that

> in the case of initiating discussions on family
> planning, religion has more effect than age:
> thus *older non-Catholic doctors* are considerably
> more active than *younger Catholic* doctors.[57]

2. *Sex.*

Surprisingly, the sex of the physician is almost never a
surveyed variable. Likewise, marital status is "underanaly-
zed."[52] Guttmacher found that while 51.1% of all respondents
"frequently prescribe contraceptive methods," 74.2% of the female specialists did so (but only 44.2% of the female general
practitioners).[53]

The preference of physicians for diaphragm over condom as
a method of choice (as high as ten to one[54]) in spite of near
equal ratings for effectiveness has been attributed to the pre-
dominance of male physicians, but we have never seen any supporting data.

3. *Urban-Rural and Regional Differences.*

Almost all the empirical data available is from geographi-
cally limited sources or does not include geographical analysis.

Guttmacher found some regional differences with the West most, and the Northeast least, receptive to contraception, but these differences can in part be understood as religious differences.[55] Spivack's research design included city-town-rural as a major variable. Introduction of the subject in the pre-marital exam was related to this variable with physicians in cities, towns and rural areas doing so "frequently" in thirty-eight, twenty-three, and twenty percent of the cases respectively.[56] Fitting of diaphragms, however, was independent of community size.

4. *Medical Specialty.*

There are considerable data revealing psycho-social differences among medical specialties. A poll in the *Medical Tribune* published in 1964 asking physicians whether abortion should be permitted for social and economic reasons showed fifty-seven percent of all physicians holding that it should be. Only forty-two percent of the obstetricians and gynecologists agreed--the lowest percentage of any specialty. (Cf. seventy-six percent of the psychiatrists agreed.)[57]

A poll of 27,741 physicians by *Modern Medicine* in 1969 revealed a similar pattern. In response to the question, "Should abortion be available to any woman capable of giving legal consent upon her own request to a competent physician?" 71.7% of the psychiatrists gave an unqualified affirmative response. This was the highest of any group except the plastic surgeons, for whom 72.6% gave a similar response. This contrasts with 41.4% of the obstetrician-gynecologists, 38.9% of the general practitioners, and 45.0% of the general surgeons.[58] If physicians are to be members of abortion review panels or to counsel women seeking abortion, there should be a much better understanding of the basis for these differences. In Chapter IV we developed the notion of the fallacy of the consensus of expert opinion. These statistics may illustrate just this phenomenon. If one were to consult the consensus of obstetricians, one would get a much different picture than if one were to consult the consensus of psychiatrists. It is possible to account for this by the greater specialized knowledge of the psychiatric

implications of unwanted pregnancy on the part of the psychiatrists, but a peculiar value constellation which led psychiatrists to select their specialty in the first place is equally
logical and perhaps a more plausible explanation. There is
little reason that the differences in technical knowledge would
account for the radical differences between general and plastic
surgeons, but very good reason to suspect that these two sub-
specialty groups have very different value constellations in
the area of the evaluation of the acceptability of surgical
procedures for personal, social, or economic reasons.

Spivack found obstetricians and gynecologists more willing
to introduce the subject of contraception in premarital exams
than general practitioners and internists (fifty to thirty-one
percent) and more likely to fit diaphragms (eighty to fifty-
eight percent).[59] Barnes *et al.* confirmed Spivack's findings
for physicians in their sample in California. Seventy-six percent of the obstetrician-gynecologists felt that physicians
should initiate family planning discussions with their patients
compared to fifty-two percent of the general practitioners.
Seventy-one percent provided IUD's in their practice compared
to thirty-seven percent of the general practitioners.[60] It is
impossible on the basis of their data to determine whether
these differences should be attributed to value differences or
differences in knowledge and experience in the field. In any
case, it is evident that specialty is an important variable.

5. *Professional vs. Lay Opinion.*

We have noted that professional specialties differ in
their attitudes and practices and that these differences may
arise from the peculiar value constellation (cultural value
complex) which led to the selection of the specialty in the
first place. It is recognized that physicians as a whole have
particular value perspectives which led them to select their
professional roles. To our knowledge, however, no comparisons
have ever been made on the subject of family planning. To the
extent that differences are related to ethical and other
evaluative aspects (the major premise primary factor) rather
than technical aspects (the minor premise primary factor) a

physician is no more qualified as an authority than a layman. The relative position of physicians with regard to the cultural value complex is as of now completely unstudied, but could provide very interesting results. We shall make an initial effort at such a comparison in Chapter VIII of this study.

E. A REVIEW OF SIGNIFICANT GAPS AND FURTHER RESEARCH FEASIBILITY

We have attempted to offer a running critique of the studies and their findings as we described them together with suggestions about the feasibility of further research. We shall briefly review our findings before going on to describe our own research.

We observed that of the few studies that consider a cultural or religious variable, "religious affiliation" or "religion" in a narrow sense is the indicator used. We argued that the cultural value complex must be measured by less rigid, more sensitive indicators. We shall use a series of scales designed to measure the cultural value complex for oral contraception as a research device.

Second, although the effect of the cultural value complex on practice is at times recognized, the effect of this complex on perception of presumably scientific (non-evaluative) facts is neither recognized nor systematically studied. We propose to use our attitude scale together with a scale which measures questions of safety, effectiveness, and demographic facts to observe relations.

The treatment of contraception by medical schools is thoroughly investigated in the A.P.H.A. study of 1964, but the effects of the very great differences are largely a matter of speculation. Such information could probably be gleaned from the unpublished data of Spivack's work and possibly from the study of the American College of Obstetrics and Gynecology. This is a particularly interesting institutional component possibly contributing to the value creation process. We shall examine the relationship of the medical school sponsorship to the cultural value complex, but a thorough study of medical education is beyond the scope of this study.

Hospitals and public health units are likewise subject to institutional pressures from political and professional bodies. Variations are well documented, but the political and cultural components of these variations have not been analyzed. Further socio-economic discrimination as seen in Hall's study of abortion remains to be documented for contraception although such discrimination seems likely.

For the other sociological variables much precise work could be done with existing unpublished data. The effect of the sex of the physician represents a particularly large gap in our knowledge as does the effect of ethnic background.

Differences between professional and lay opinion on the non-scientific aspects of family planning constitute the last specific area of needed research we shall mention. It is reasonable to assume that the unique sociological characteristics of the professional medical subgroups give rise to significant differences such as their often mentioned conservatism. We shall extend the use of our cultural value complex scales to a group of patients to test this relationship.

Finally we must observe that none of the studies we have mentioned have been particularly statistically oriented. Generally the effect of a socio-cultural variable is measured by means of a bi-polar division of a particular attitudinal or behavioural characteristic. Thus Catholic vs. non-Catholic or under forty-five vs. over forty-five are used as categories. It would be valuable to think in terms of even zero-sum correlation coefficients for such factors. Our first task in the empirical study is the initial construction of the cultural value complex scales. This shall be undertaken in the next chapter.

[1]Mary Jean Cornish, Florence Ruderman, and Sydney S. Spivack, *Doctors and Family Planning* (New York: National Committee on Maternal Health, Inc., 1963), p. 25 (italics added). The data are taken from the most substantial study of physicians' attitudes on family planning, which was done at the Bureau of Applied Social Research at Columbia University. Spivack was the designer and executer of the study and we shall frequently refer to him in citing further conclusions.

[2]*Ibid.*, p. 36, note 5.

[3]Here we consider abortion, sterilization, hormonal steroids, and the intra-uterine device to be the most effective.

[4]Freedman devotes only one brief paragraph to the subject and cites only the Spivack study. See Ronald Freedman, "The Sociology of Human Fertility: A Trend Report and Bibliography," *Current Sociology*, XI, No. 2 (1962), p. 64.

[5]Cornish, *Doctors and Family Planning*, p. 23.

[6]A. J. Cunningham, "Physicians and Contraception," *Canadian Medical Association Journal*, XCII (January 9, 1965), p. 87.

[7]Gordon W. Perkin, "Physicians and Contraception," *Canadian Medical Association Journal*, XCII (March 20, 1965), p. 632. The exchange was stimulated by an editorial, "Physicians and Contraception," *Canadian Medical Association Journal*, XCI (October 11, 1964), pp. 820-21. The fact that Cunningham is impressed with the possibility of a post-fertilization action of oral contraceptives while Perkin argues "there has been no evidence to indicate that fertilization of an ovum occurs" is undoubtedly also being influenced by cultural level factors.

[8]Cornish, *Doctors and Family Planning*, p. 19.

[9]Cornelius C. Bakker and Cameron R. Dightman, "Physicians and Family Planning: A Persistent Ambivalence," *Obstetrics and Gynecology*, XXV (February, 1965), p. 282.

[10]Bakker and Dightman, "Physicians and Family Planning," p. 282. The effect of medical education will be discussed later.

[11]Cornish, *Doctors and Family Planning*, p. 4. For the premarital exam only twenty-two percent initiate discussion "very frequently." The remainder do so "often" (eleven percent) or "occasionally" (twenty percent). For the postpartum exam only twenty-seven percent initiate discussion "almost always," twenty-three percent "sometimes." Other studies give similar data.

See E. M. Nash, "Attitudes of Physicians Affecting Contraceptive Practice," in *Manual of Contraceptive Practice*, ed. by Marry S. Calderone (Baltimore: Williams and Wilkins, 1964), p. 97. Here thirty-seven percent were found to "routinely" make suggestions in the premarital exam with another twenty-eight percent doing so "only if specifically requested." Only eleven percent did so "routinely" in the postpartum exam.

For physicians in the study of Siegel and Dillehay, 35.7% initiated discussions of family planning. Another 28.6% discussed the subject if the family introduced the subject; 17.9% refused to discuss it or found "no occasion" to. Earl Siegel and Ronald C. Dillehay, "Some Approaches to Family Planning Counseling in Local Health Departments: A Survey of Public Health Nurses and Physicians," *American Journal of Public Health*, LVI (November, 1966), p. 1843.

[12] John Barnes, Larry Johnson, Helen Kaufman, William Nichols, and Peter Olsson, "Attitudes and Practices of Physicians Concerning Birth Control in Two California Counties," 1965 (unpublished manuscript).

[13] Nash, "Attitudes," p. 98. Also see C. N. Herndon and E. M. Nash, "Premarriage and Marriage Counselling: A Study of Practices of North Carolina Physicians," *Journal of the American Medical Association* (May 5, 1962), p. 395, and Lee Rainwater, *And the Poor Get Children* (Chicago: Quadrangle Books, 1960).

[14] Joseph J. Spengler, "Values and Fertility Analysis," *Demography*, II, No. 1 (1966), p. 119.

[15] Spengler attacks Kunkel for taking this view. *Ibid.*, p. 113. Spengler himself seems to be ambivalent with regard to value system changes being initiators of changes in preference systems which in turn are responsible for changes in demographic behavior. *Ibid.*, pp. 128-29. Easterlin's economic analysis of the American baby boom seems critical of value interpretations. Nevertheless preference system changes seen in the rural-urban shift and the migratory shift from Southeastern to Northwestern Europe are central to his argument. See Richard Easterlin, *The American Baby Boom in Historical Perspective* (n.p.: National Bureau of Economic Research, 1962).

[16] Cornish, *Doctors and Family Planning*, p. 48.

[17] *Ibid.*, p. 71.

[18] The Eliot study of hospitals and the Tietze study of medical schools are also sensitive to this variable as are most of the large scale studies of laymen.

[19] Charles J. McFadden, *Medical Ethics* (Philadelphia: F. A. Davis Company, 1956), p. 100.

[20] Cornish, *Doctors and Family Planning*, p. 31.

[21] *Ibid.*, p. 33.

[22]Cornish, *Doctors and Family Planning*, p. 31.

[23]*Ibid.*, pp. 36-37.

[24]Barnes, *et al.*, Part VI, p. 3.

[25]*Ibid.*, p. 4.

[26]Cornish, *Doctors and Family Planning*, p. 59.

[27]Lake, "The Pill," p. 174.

[28]Eliot and Meier, "Fertility Control," p. 588.

[29]*Ibid.*, pp. 583, 586.

[30]AMA Committee on Human Reproduction [Report of], "The Control of Fertility," *Journal of the American Medical Association*, CXCIV, No. 4 (October 25, 1965), p. 462. Also see H. C. Wood, "Medical Responsibility in Solving Population Problems," *Pacific Medicine and Surgery*, LCCIV (July-August, 1966), p. 244.

[31]Cornish, *Doctors and Family Planning*, p. 53. A Catholic had a 65% chance of getting one from a non-Catholic doctor, but this probably does not indicate a value conflict. Cornish observes that Catholics wanting contraceptive advice probably avoid the Catholic physician. Eliot notes that referrals are not even permitted in some Catholic hospitals in spite of the fact that in some cases the majority of the patients may be non-Catholic and "many [indigent] patients did not choose the hospital, but were assigned to it." Eliot and Meier, "Fertility Control," p. 586.

[32]Tietze, "Teaching of Fertility Regulation," p. 21.

[33]Harold I. Lief, "Orientation of Future Physicians in Psycho-sexual Attitudes," *Manual of Contraceptive Practice*, p. 105.

[34]See J. R. Willson, "The Physician's Responsibility in Family Planning and Population Control," *Michigan Medicine*, LXIV (May, 1965), p. 333; C. L. Buxton, "The Doctor's Responsibility in Population Control," *Northwest Medicine*, LXV (February, 1966), p. 113; Eliot and Meier, "Fertility Control," p. 588; Nash, "Attitudes," p. 102; Bakker and Dightman, "Physicians and Family Planning," pp. 280, 282; Guttmacher, "Conception Control," pp. 4, 10; Cornish, *Doctors and Family Planning*, pp. 36-37.

[35]Guttmacher, "Conception Control," p. 4.

[36]Tietze, "Teaching of Fertility Regulation," pp. 20, 22-23.

[37]Eliot and Meier, "Fertility Control," pp. 582-91.

[38]Eliot and Meier, "Fertility Control," pp. 582-91.

[39]Hall, "Therapeutic Abortion," p. 518.

[40]*Ibid.*, p. 531.

[41]Siegel and Dillehay, "Family Planning Counseling," p. 1841.

[42]*Ibid.*, p. 1842. This combines those categories where the "professional only" initiates and "sometimes family, sometimes professional." For physicians the percentages were 35.7 and 0 respectively. For nurses they were 27.6 and 26.2

[43]Eliot, *et al.*, "Michigan Physicians' Views."

[44]This is in spite of the official A.P.H.A. resolution "that federal, state, and local governments include family planning as an integral part of their health program." See Gordon W. Perkin, "Physicians and Contraception," p. 632. Also see Governing Council of A.P.H.A., "Policy Statements: The Population Problem," *American Journal of Public Health*, IL (December, 1959), pp. 1703-04.

[45]Bakker and Dightman, "Physicians and Family Planning," p. 280.

[46]Eliot, *et al.*, "Michigan Physicians' Views."

[47]Barnes, *et al.*, "Attitudes and Practices of Physicians," Part VI, pp. 7-9.

[48]"Modern Medicine Poll," p. 21.

[49]Guttmacher, "Conception Control," p. 8.

[50]Cornish, *Doctors and Family Planning*, p. 32. Also see the data of Nash, "Attitudes of Physicians," p. 98.

[51]Cornish, *Doctors and Family Planning*, p. 49.

[52]Siegel and Dillehay not only note differences between physicians and public health nurses (which could be accounted for in many ways), but also between nurses who had children and those who did not. Siegel and Dillehay, "Family Planning Counseling," p. 1943.

[53]Guttmacher, "Fertility Control," p. 8. Unfortunately Guttmacher does not give sufficient information for legitimate comparison. We are not told what percentage of all specialists "frequently prescribe contraceptive methods."

[54]See Nash, "Attitudes of Physicians," p. 100.

[55]Guttmacher, "Fertility Control," p. 6.

[56] Cornish, *Doctors and Family Planning*, p. 47. This confirms Guttmacher's findings; Guttmacher, "Fertility Control," p. 8.

[57] "Social, Economic Basis for Abortion Upheld," p. 21.

[58] "Modern Medicine Poll," p. 19.

[59] Cornish, *Doctors and Family Planning*, p. 42.

[60] Barnes, *et al.*, "Attitudes and Practices of Physicians," Part VI, pp. 9-14.

CHAPTER VI

THE BIRTH CONTROL CULTURAL VALUE COMPLEX

> The regulation of conception appears necessary for
> many couples who wish to achieve a responsible,
> open and reasonable parenthood in today's circum-
> stances. If they are to observe and cultivate
> all the essential values of marriage, married
> people need decent and human means for the regu-
> lation of conception.
>
> --Majority Papal Commission Report, 1966

> Since husbands and wives owe a responsibility to
> other families on the earth, they must take into
> account the relation of natural resources to the
> total population. Under present circumstances
> this means that most couples have not only the
> right but also the moral obligation to space and
> limit the number of births.
>
> --Mansfield Report, 1959

> Was not the world created only for propagation?
>
> --Talmud (Hagiga 2b)

While religion is probably the best sociological measure
for predicting decisions made about birth control, there is
evidence that it is not to be equated with the complex of
values from which decisions are made. We saw in Chapter V that
very few studies of physicians' attitudes and practices related
to oral contraception, or birth control more generally, even
measured religion as a major variable. None went beyond this
gross sociological measure to examine the actual ethical and
other values of the physicians. In Chapter VII we shall report
evidence that the relationship between religious affiliation
and evaluation of contraception is far from perfect. In order
to do this it is necessary to develop the dimensions of evaluation of contraception, what in Chapter IV we called the "cultural value complex." Our method for developing these dimensions will be drawn in modified form from the structural anthropologists who have developed the techniques of content
analysis.[1]

Claude Lévi-Strauss, in an essay on "The Structural Study
of Myth," has demonstrated that in addition to the social and

185

historical study of the context of complex symbolic religious
phenomena such as myth, much insight can be gained by examining
the content and structure of the symbolic constructions themselves.[2] He observes that in spite of myths being collected in
widely different regions and circumstances, there is an "as-
tounding similarity" among them. He asks a troubling question
to social relativists who have been brought up on the belief
that a social phenomenon can be fully explained and has been
fully analyzed when its historical origin and context has been
described. Drawing from the science of linguistics he argues
that myth, like the rest of language, is made up of constituent
units. The units of myth, however, differ from the rest of
language in that they belong to a "higher and more complex order." These are found "on the sentence level." He calls them
the "gross constituent units."[3] The method used in the analysis of content and structure is the breaking down of the myth
into the shortest possible sentences (gross constituent units),
writing each on an index card which can be physically moved
during the analysis.[4]

We have argued in Chapter IV that the cultural value complex includes an objectively legitimated component which can be
understood as being religious. We suggest that while there are
many obvious differences there are also many similarities between myths and cultural value complexes. Myths are complex
symbolic formulations attempting to represent certain patterns
of meaning. They, so the structuralist says, are attempts to
symbolically resolve basic dilemmas about the meaning of existence. In terms of the unified theory of action, they are specific symbolic formulations in the cultural sphere of patterns
of existential meaning. By analogy we suggest that cultural
value complexes are specific symbolic formulations in the cultural sphere of evaluative symbolization. To be sure, the cultural value complex for birth control is less rigidly formulated than the typical myth, but myths also exist in many versions and variations. Lévi-Strauss argues that a myth consists
not of a standard "authentic" version and many variants, but in
the totality of the versions:

> Our method thus eliminates a problem which has, so
> far, been one of the main obstacles to the progress
> of mythological studies, namely, the quest for the
> true version, or the earlier one. On the contrary,
> we define the myth as consisting of all its ver-
> sions....An important consequence follows. If a
> myth is made up of all its variants, structural
> analysis should take all of them into account.[5]

We propose a similar undertaking for the construction of a
cultural value complex. In this chapter we shall report the
results of a sentence by sentence analysis of official pronouncements on birth control and birth control related subjects
by as many religious groups as we have been able to obtain. It
has been necessary to limit the accumulation of "data" in several ways. First we are looking at religious groups because we
are interested primarily in the ethical and other evaluative
dimensions, not the pharmacological and other technical dimensions which might receive attention in pronouncements by medical groups. We have limited ourselves to what we have called
"official" pronouncements by which we mean statements made on
behalf of some religious group rather than statements of individual views.[6] It is our working hypothesis that analysis of a
sufficient number of sufficiently diverse documents of this
type will provide a working list of the dimensions of evaluation of an issue area which taken together make up the cultural
value complex. The homogeneity of the dimensions isolated
through this technique will then be tested empirically in the
study which will be discussed in the next chapter.

We have further limited the pronouncements to those of
religious groups whose membership includes Americans and those
written in the period from 1930 to the present. These limitations are compatible with the composition of the group of physicians we shall be studying. In all we have accumulated a
collection of seventy-four statements which have been used in
this analysis. We do not claim that this is a complete list.
We have attempted to obtain a representative sample stressing
diversity of positions. A full list of the statements we have
used is presented in Appendix VI.

Before proceeding with the analysis we should make clear
two things we shall not be doing. First, we shall not

undertake a comparative study of the positions of different
religious groups on the subject of birth control. In fact we
shall be using statements which reveal that the birth control
cultural value complex is indeed very complex, that there are
often differences within denominational groups which are very
basic. Rather, our task is to attempt to isolate the dimensions of evaluation which run throughout the collection of
statements. Second, we shall not provide an account of the
historical development of the positions of various groups.[7]
Both of these tasks are interesting and worthwhile, but beyond
the scope of the present project.

We began with a unit by unit analysis of six statements
which we selected on the basis of their being major, detailed
statements which in most cases have had an important influence
on the literature in the field. We selected statements representative of a broad spectrum of positions and from different
points over the time period we are studying.[8]

Beginning with these six statements we coded each sentence
or discrete phrase according to the categories developed in
Chapters II through IV of this study. Treating each sentence
or phrase as a "gross constituent unit," we classified the
units as examples of cognitive, expressive, evaluative, and
existential meaning symbolization. (See Chapter II and Figure
4 for further discussion of these categories.) There were some
statements of meaning grounding (particularly in the more theologically oriented documents) and expressions of cathexis for,
or identification with, certain groups, but, as might be expected, most of the units were either statements of evaluation
or statements of beliefs about the non-evaluative facts. We
shall concern ourselves primarily with the latter which we, in
Chapter IV, identified as the primary factors in the decision-
making process.

Following this initial classification of the units, we
then went back through the units which were statements of evaluation and attempted to classify them further on the basis of
the dimensions of evaluation as discussed in Chapter III and
Figure 5. In many cases the units could not be further classified. For instance, in the 1961 "Statement on Birth Control,"

approved by the conservative Jewish Committee on Jewish Law and Standards, it says:

> Where birth control is to be practiced, it is preferable that the woman use the contraceptive. It is the woman who bears the hardships incidental to childbirth; it is, in other words, her condition primarily which creates the justification for interfering with conception.[9]

The key term which identifies this series of statements as evaluative is "preferable." A strict reading of the text, however, does not give us any basis for conclusively determining that the committee is claiming that it is *morally* preferable although the context implies this to be the case.

We shall refrain from speculating about the exact references for evaluative terms limiting our analysis to situations where the meaning of the text is spelled out. We shall label an evaluation "moral" only when the unit contains explicit moral terminology or has all the characteristics of a moral statement as discussed in Chapter III.

A. MORAL DIMENSIONS

Among the statements which were classified as evaluative and contained sufficient specificity to identify as representing the various dimensions of evaluation, there was an overwhelming proportion of moral statements. This is what we might expect from the type of statements being analyzed. From the initial six statements we formed tentative hypotheses about the themes in the moral factor of the cultural value complex. These were then tested, corroborated, and modified by analysis of the remaining sixty-eight statements. The result was that we identified five major themes which appeared as moral factors in the cultural value complex.

1. *General Moral Statements.*

First, we found many statements which could clearly be identified as moral statements, but could not be further classified as providing any basis for the moral claim. While these statements give us the least information about what the moral

judgments are, they are the most inclusive. They would presumably be affirmed or rejected by any one sharing the moral
judgment about birth control regardless of the reasons for his
judgment. The 1931 statement by the Federal Council of
Churches was an important document because it was the first
major endorsement by an American religious body following the
explosion of the birth control issue in 1930 with the Roman
encyclical, *Casti Connubii*, and the Anglican limited endorsement of birth control at the 1930 Lambeth Conference. In the
Federal Council of Churches statement the majority of the committee drafting the statement reached the conclusion that "the
careful and constrained use of contraceptives by married people
is valid and moral."[10]

Although they go on to spell out reasons for their moral
judgment, this initial summary statement is obviously very general. Presumably it could be subscribed to by anyone approving
of birth control on moral grounds regardless of what the
grounds were although some would go beyond this cautious endorsement.

The minority of the committee expressed moral doubts about
the practice of birth control, appealing to the norm of abstinence. Their equally general moral judgment was:

> In view of the wisespread doubt among Christian
> people of the morality of the use of contracep-
> tives, and the scruples experienced by many in
> making use of them, it appears to these members
> of the committee to be the plain duty of the
> Christian Church, when control of conception is
> necessary, to uphold the standard of abstinence
> as the ideal....[11]

The Conservative Jewish "Statement on Birth Control," in a
review of the Jewish tradition, offers a general moral judgment
favoring birth control without specifying the conditions or
reasons for the judgment claiming "...in some circumstances it
was considered morally right to curtail childbirth."[12]

In some statements we have examined the claims of the
moral judgment went beyond the simple statement of moral approval or disapproval giving a hint of the subthemes, but still
not giving sufficient information to identify the nature of the
moral argument. The 1962 General Conference of the Evangelical

United Brethren Church passed a resolution on responsible
parenthood which included the statement that:

> Within marriage, it is ethically and morally right
> to properly use methods and techniques, medically
> approved, for the purpose of achieving planned
> and responsible parenthood.[13]

This statement gives us hints of some of the reasons for
their judgment of moral approval. The purpose is the achievement of responsible parenthood and the approval is limited to
use within marriage, but the argument is still not made explicit. We included some of these general statements of moral approval and disapproval in a "general morality" subscale in our
empirical study of the cultural value complex of physicians
which we shall report in the next chapter. This will serve as
a control so that we are assured that we have not excluded any
who morally disapprove or approve of birth control for reasons
other than the ones encompassing the specific themes we shall
operationalize in the other subscales.

2. *Birth Control and Promiscuity.*

We have argued that it is a common but oversimplified assumption that the issue of birth control can be understood as
one in which Catholics line up on one side and non-Catholics
on the other. It is equally oversimplified to maintain that
the basis for the moral judgments about birth control is related to the distinction between natural and artificial means of
contraception. We shall examine this theme below: it is only
one among several factors and, judging from both the Catholic
and non-Catholic statements we have examined, clearly not the
most important factor.

While it is recognized that some Catholics, particularly
recently, have overall moral judgments favoring the practice of
birth control, it is not so often realized that many non-
Catholics have moral reservations about its practice. We shall
illustrate this observation throughout the remaining four
themes which we shall explore. We had a hint of the non-
Catholic reservations in the statements quoted above in the
minority position of the Federal Council of Churches and in the

Evangelical United Brethren position. The judgment of ethical
rightness was limited to practice "within marriage." If Catholics disapprove of certain methods of birth control for their
"unnaturalness," certain non-Catholic groups, especially more
conservative Protestant denominations, are worried about en-
dorsing birth control because they feel that it will inevitably
lead to an increase in sexual relations outside marriage which
they find morally wrong.

In the important statement on "Responsible Parenthood and
the Population Problem" of the Council for Christian Social Action adopted in January of 1960, the reservations about promiscuity are explicit:

> Christians are deeply concerned about the moral
> problems of sex relations before marriage, and
> outside of the marriage bond. From the Christian
> viewpoint both are violations of God's will as
> expressed in the moral law. Advocacy of the use
> of contraceptives by married couples is not an
> endorsement of promiscuity among the unmarried.[14]

Similar reservations are expressed in the statement of the
Augustana Evangelical Lutheran Church in 1954 in which it was
said:

> Sex relations outside of marriage, whether before
> an intended marriage or outside an established
> marriage bond, are a violation of God's will.
> The use of contraceptives by the unmarried can
> indeed reduce the risk of an illegitimate child,
> but this changes the character of premarital
> relationships just as little as the fact that
> one party to adultery may be sterile changes
> the nature of adultery.[15]

Concern with the possibility of increasing sexual activity
outside of the marital bond is not limited to the Protestant
churches. Pope Paul, in his encyclical, *Humanae Vitae*, but-
tresses his other arguments against "artificial birth control"
with the following statement:

> Upright men can even better convince themselves of
> the solid grounds on which the teaching of the
> Church in this field is based, if they care to re-
> flect upon the consequences of methods of artifi-
> cial birth control. Let them consider, first of
> all, how wide and easy a road would thus be opened
> up towards conjugal infidelity and the general
> lowering of morality.[16]

The themes we are developing relating to the morality of contraception are not simple. In each case moral claims are made both favoring and opposing the practice of contraception. In the case of the promiscuity theme, however, it is seldom that an argument is offered that premarital sexual relations are morally right. It is somewhat more plausible, however, to argue that one has a moral obligation to practice contraception if one is involved in premarital sexual relations. To our knowledge no religious group has formally made such an argument. Two lines of argument were found, however, which lead to positions related to the promiscuity theme which favor the availability of contraception. One is to deny that the availability of contraceptives will lead to lowered standards of morality related to promiscuity. The Reformed Church in America in a 1960 statement endorsed by the General Synod said:

> The argument that available contraceptives will lead to an increased sexual immorality is dubious. If the availability of contraceptives will cause the church to develop a more positive expression of sex morality and a positive program of training in the values of chastity and marital fidelity it may prove a blessing.[17]

The other development has been the gradual elimination of the qualification of marital status from statement of approval of birth control practices and the dissemination of birth control information. In the most recent Methodist statement on responsible parenthood, the Board of Christian Social Concerns calls upon the church and "our common society" to "make information and materials available so *all* can exercise responsible choice in the area of conception control."[18]

In the next chapter we shall incorporate a subscale in our empirical study of physicians which attempts to measure the theme of the morality of contraception in relation to promiscuity.

3. *Moral Obligations and the Ends of Marriage.*

A third theme identified as part of the moral factor in the cultural value complex deals with the "ends of marriage." This is also a complex moral theme ranging from the moral requirement to make every act a procreative possibility to a moral obligation to avoid procreation in certain circumstances. Probably the position most opposed to contraception based on the theme of the ends of marriage is that of the Orthodox Church. One recent article stating the Orthodox position said simply, "The birth of children is the principal aim of marriage." The article called the Lambeth Conference of 1958, which had endorsed contraception, "a betrayal of Christian moral principles."[19]

Archbishop Michael of the Greek Archdiocese of North and South America, in perhaps the strongest moral condemnation of birth control ever officially issued by a religious group with American members, maintained in a 1956 statement:

> If wedded couples have sexual intercourse only as a means of satisfaction for their carnal desires, then the Sacrament of Matrimony--"this great Mystery," as the Apostle Paul terms it--loses its value and its holy purpose and deteriorates into a means of sexual satisfaction. In other words, the union of the partners blessed by the Church is thus changed to respectable immorality.
> If husband and wife do not desire to have many children, they ought to abstain from all conjugal relations until they are able to have many children, and then come together again in sexual union relying entirely and solely on God's omniscience.
> The use of contraceptive devices for the prevention of childbirth is forbidden and condemned unreservedly by the Greek Orthodox Church.[20]

The Roman Catholic pronouncements relating to the ends of marriage reveal many similarities to the Orthodox position, but their argument is very complex in detail. Substantial diversity exists within the contemporary Catholic literature. In *Casti Connubii*, the major document of the period prior to the recent papal commission and the encyclical *Humanae Vitae*, Pius XI defended the moral primacy of the procreative function:

> But no reason, however grave, may be put forward by which anything *intrinsically* against nature may become conformable to nature and morally good. Since, therefore, *the conjugal act* is destined primarily *by nature* for the begetting of children, those who in exercising it deliberately frustrate its natural power and purpose sin against nature and commit a deed which is shameful and *intrinsically vicious*....[21]

John T. Noonan, however, points out that "the admission of multiple purposes in marital intercourse has been a commonplace of Catholic theology since the seventeenth century."[22] He reports that several efforts were made by conservative theologians to induce Vatican II to assert that procreation was the primary end of marriage and that these were rejected.[23] The final document of Vatican II, "The Constitution of the Church in the Modern World," speaks of the unity of marriage as one of its ends. "Married love," it says, "is uniquely expressed and perfected by the exercise of the acts proper to marriage."[24] Likewise, Paul VI, in *Humanae Vitae*, speaks of the two meanings of the conjugal acts: the unitive and the procreative.[25]

With the general Catholic acceptance of the multiple ends of marriage there are still two differences which are very important. The first is whether every sexual act must have the potential of both ends in order to be moral. The papal commission majority report says it does not:

> ...the morality of sexual acts between married people takes its meaning first of all and specifically from the ordering of their actions in a fruitful married life, that is one which is practiced with responsible, generous and prudent parenthood. It does not depend upon the direct fecundity of each and every particular act.[26]

In contrast, *Humanae Vitae* insists that for the unitive and procreative ends of marriage there is an "inseparable connection, willed by God and unable to be broken by man on his own initiative." It claims that according to the natural law "every marriage act...must remain open to the transmission of life."[27]

The second difference is the degree to which the procreative end is seen as including a responsibility for the raising and educating of children. If the moral responsibility of marriage includes the educating of offspring, then some practice of birth control may be morally tolerable or even required. While *Humanae Vitae* is silent on educational implications in its discussion of the procreative end of marriage, Vatican II and the Papal Commission's majority report emphasize the educative aspect. According to Vatican II, "Marriage and conjugal

love by their nature are ordered to the procreation and education of offspring."[28] The majority report says that couples
have a moral responsibility of responsible parenthood for which
"they will make a judgment in conscience before God about the
number of children to have and educate."[29]

Though the non-Catholic statements generally place more
emphasis on the non-procreative aspects of marital obligation,
they, too, show considerable range in their understanding of
the ends of marriage. The Committee on Jewish Law and Standards has endorsed a statement saying, "God created the world
to be a home for human life, and it is incumbent on man and
woman to further God's plan by procreating, by bringing children into the world and raising them to continue the work of
creation."[30] A 1960 statement of the Central Conference of
American Rabbis has a somewhat different tone. It says, "We
believe that it is the sacred duty of married couples to 'be
fruitful and multiply,'" but adds that "a righteous God does
not require the unlimited birth of children who may by unfavor-
able social and economic circumstances be denied a chance for a
decent and wholesome life."[31]

Many Protestant groups also speak of the two ends of marriage, the Lambeth Conference of 1958 calling procreation "a
primary obligation of Christian marriage." They emphasize the
non-procreative obligations, however. The Lambeth Conference
said responsible parenthood "built on obedience to all the
duties of marriage, requires a wise stewardship of the resources and abilities of the family...."[32] Several Protestant
groups follow the implications of the non-procreative ends of
marriage to their logical conclusion claiming that there is a
moral obligation to practice contraception. The General Assembly of the Presbyterian Church in the United States in 1960
said:

> The God whose creative grace makes possible the
> blessing of children through marriage likewise
> vests man and wife with moral responsibility in
> the exercise of their procreative function....The
> responsibility of prospective parents obligates
> them to consider well how their children are to
> be provided with that which will make for their
> best physical, cultural, moral and spiritual de-
> velopment.[33]

4. *Obligations Related to Naturalness and Artificiality.*

Casti Connubii speaks of those who "deliberately frustrate the natural power" of the conjugal act as "sinning against nature."[34] Pope Paul, in *Humanae Vitae*, distinguishes between rhythm in which "the married couple make legitimate use of a natural disposition" and using means directly contrary to fecundation which impede "the development of a natural process."[35]

The Rabbinical Alliance of America, representing the viewpoint of Orthodox Judaism, stated, "Orthodox Judaism does not condone any artificial birth control measures by the male spouse under any circumstances."[36] They do, however, endorse female measures where the health of the woman is jeopardized.

Protestant statements tend to either ignor or directly attack the distinction between natural and artificial means. The Evangelical and Reformed Church in 1960 claimed that "there is no moral distinction between the so-called 'rhythm method' of averting conception and the responsible use of artificial barriers...."[37] The Reformed Church in America in 1962 went even further. They said that responsible parenthood (and from the context it is clear they mean contraception other than rhythm) is the "readiest, most natural way of perpetuating and extending the Kingdom of God."[38]

5. *Moral Obligations Related to Population Growth.*

Virtually every statement we have examined reflects the intimate link between contraception and population growth. This is the fifth and last theme we have identified in the moral dimensions of the birth control cultural value complex. The Mansfield Report of the World Council of Churches Ecumenical Study Group is typical. Called "Responsible Parenthood and the Population Problem," it begins with an account of the "crisis" the world is experiencing from the rapid growth of population. The Episcopal Church in 1961 said that "...warnings against the explosive results of world population increase... have raised with new urgency questions of the morality of restricting population growth through birth control measures and planned parenthood...."[39] The same statement by the Presbyterian Church of the U.S. quoted above to the effect that God vests man and wife with moral responsibility in the exercise of their procreative functions goes on to say "this responsibility is intensified today by what is known as 'the population explosion' and the threats to human welfare it involves."[40]

Not all religious groups, however, consider the pressures of population growth to be a basis for the moral justification or obligation to practice birth control. Judaism, as reflected in the Conservative Committee on Jewish Law and Standards, holds that in extreme circumstances it is considered morally justified to curtail birth. However, the *Jewish* population, according to their reading of the data, is far from being endangered by overpopulation. Pointing to the loss of "a third" of its members as a result of Nazi persecution and extermination, they observe that they are under a "divine imperative to serve as a witness of the Torah." "A decimated Jewish people," they say, "is an impaired tool in the divine service."[41]

The Catholic position as seen in papal pronouncements is to recognize the existence of a threat from rapid population growth,[42] but to claim that this is not sufficient reason to violate one's moral obligation to God and family. In *Mater et Magistra*, Pope John XXIII wrote:

> Hence, the real solution of the problem (over-population) is not to be found in expedients which offend against the divinely established moral order or which attack human life at its very source, but in a renewed, scientific and technical effort on man's part to deepen and extend his dominion over nature....[43]

Thus the population theme, like the others, has potential moral claims both supporting and rejecting the use of contraception. In our empirical study we shall develop these five themes (general moral evaluation, promiscuity, the ends of marriage, the naturalness of contraception, and population) into subscales of the moral factor of the cultural value complex.

B. OTHER DIMENSIONS

In Chapter III we outlined personal, group referential, and legal bases of legitimation of evaluation as well as types of objective legitimation other than the moral. Probably none

of these other dimensions plays as significant a role as the
moral in the evaluation of contraception. Of these the dimension of personal pleasure or usefulness is probably the most
significant.

It is quite possible that one could find the practice of
birth control perfectly moral, but unpleasant for one reason or
another. On the other hand, contraception may be evaluated as
making life more pleasurable or convenient or easier from a
personal point of view, but wrong from a moral point of view.
Some of the statements we have examined, both Protestant[44] and
Catholic,[45] speak of the pleasures and joys of procreation.
Presumably a person who views the production of offspring as
one of the great personal pleasures of life would tend to eval-
uate contraception in a somewhat different way from one who
finds children a perpetual nuisance. Likewise personal pleasure and satisfaction can be seen as being derived from the
practice of contraception.[46] Different methods of contraception may be evaluated differently from the standpoint of personal pleasure even though they are seen as morally equivalent.
The Council for Christian Social Action of the United Church of
Christ statement on "Responsible Parenthood and the Population
Problem," maintains that "the *means* of family planning are in
large measure matters of clinical and aesthetic choice."[47]

The evaluation of contraception with reference to personal
pleasure, convenience, and satisfaction (i.e., evaluation which
is personally legitimated) may have complex origins. Dissatisfaction with certain methods such as the diaphragm on the
grounds of personal displeasure may be rooted directly in the
dislike of the technique itself or the displeasure may be the
result of a moral judgment. Furthermore, personally legitimated evaluations may be rooted in beliefs about the non-evaluative facts. Some may believe that taking the birth control
pill may be unpleasant because of unpleasant side effects anticipated. Others may find it unpleasant because of the nuisance
of having to take a pill every day, while still others may anticipate displeasure derivatively because of a negative moral
judgment. We shall incorporate a scale designed to measure
evaluations based on personal pleasure and convenience of oral

contraception in our empirical study. We shall examine the
results to see if such evaluations are more closely related to
moral judgments or beliefs about the non-evaluative facts.

The remaining dimensions of evaluation appear to play a
minor role in the evaluation of contraception. There was little evidence of evaluation which was based on reference to loyalty to particular groups of which an individual is a member.
This is not to say, of course, that group identification and
loyalty does not play an important role in influencing the
other dimensions of evaluation. This means only that evaluations of contraception are not legitimated or *justified* as being "the way our group does things" the way table manners or
other folkways might be. Rather they are justified in moral
terms (or as matters of personal preference).

A few of the earlier statements we examined referred to
the legality of contraception, but these were offering arguments (based primarily on moral grounds) why the law should be
changed, occasionally combined with the implication that one
has a moral obligation to follow a particular practice because
it is required by civil law. The 1960 Evangelical and Reformed
Church action of the General Council is an example. Concluding
that they were "convinced of the moral soundness of wise and
responsible birth-control," they called

> attention to the fact that those who seek such
> information for immoral reasons apparently have
> little difficulty in securing it, while under
> present legal restraints, many who need and wish
> such information for good moral reasons find it
> difficult if not impossible to secure it from
> sources to which they are restricted by self-
> respect and Christian conscience.[48]

Since the Supreme Court decision in *Griswold v. Connecticut* in 1965, this has become an even less significant basis for
evaluation with the possible exception of a few localities
where prescribing contraceptives for unmarried women remains
illegal even if such legal provisions are routinely ignored by
most physicians.

There are categories of evaluation in the cultural value
complex which are legitimated by reference to a standard more
universal than personal preferences, group patterns, or legal

provisions of the civil law. Of the "objectively legitimated" categories of evaluation certainly the moral dominates the contraception cultural value complex. We have already treated this in detail. The value of Truth or knowledge for its own sake may play an important role in decisions about undertaking research to develop new contraceptive technologies (although other, more utilitarian reasons also play an important role in those decisions). We, however, will be examining physician decision-making in a clinical context. This dimension seems to play a minor role at most in clinical decisions.

It is important to separate aesthetics as an objectively legitimated value from matters of personal taste. We have already cited one statement which said that selection of the means of family planning includes the dimension of aesthetic choice, but suggested that this was being used in a way which made it clear that the authors were referring to personally legitimated evaluation. Contraceptive techniques have not gained the status of the symphony or of great painting. Aesthetic judgment in this sense appears to play a minor role in contraceptive decision-making.

Finally there are values which we have called orientational which form the link between evaluational and meaning grounding symbolization. The themes of man's relationship to nature and to time have appeared upon occasion in the statements we have examined. Fortunately, the work of Kluckhohn and Strodtbeck has developed the themes of the orientational values in detail on the basis of substantial empirical cross-cultural study.[49] We shall incorporate a few items attempting to measure these orientational values into our empirical study. We have already discussed these themes in Chapter III.

This completes our survey of church statements on birth control and birth control related matters. In our empirical study we shall include five themes which are part of the moral evaluation (general moral judgments, promiscuity, the ends of marriage, the naturalness of contraception, and demographic factors), the dimension of personal pleasure and preferences, and a small number of items drawn from the work of Kluckhohn and Strodtbeck which attempt to measure the orientational values.

NOTES

CHAPTER VI

[1]See Claude Lévi-Strauss, "The Structural Study of Myth,"
in *Structural Anthropology* (Garden City, N.Y.: Doubleday and
Company, 1963), pp. 202-28, and Edmund Leach, "Lévi-Strauss in
the Garden of Eden: An Examination of Some Recent Developments
in the Analysis of Myth," in *Reader in Comparative Religion: An
Anthropological Approach*, second edition, ed. by William A.
Lessa and Evon Z. Vogt (New York: Harper and Row, 1965), pp.
574-81.

[2]Some of the structuralists' most provacative and controversial work comes from the analysis of the patterns of relationship among the units of the myth. This task is intertwined
with the examination of the content of the units in which
themes such as autochthonous origin and denial of autochthonous
origin of man, life and death, and nature and culture (the raw
and the cooked) are abstracted. Both of these enterprises can
be applied to the study of the cultural value complex. The analysis of the patterns of relationship among the units could be
carried out on the cultural value complex. We anticipate that
the analogy would be sustained. We plan such an undertaking
in the future for the statements we have collected related to
birth control, but this would take us far beyond the needs of
the present. We shall limit ourselves primarily to the use of
the structuralist methodology for the isolation and abstraction
of major themes (what we have called the dimensions of evaluation).

[3]Lévi-Strauss, "The Structural Study of Myth," pp. 203-7.

[4]*Ibid.*, p. 207.

[5]*Ibid.*, p. 213.

[6]This was necessary to put some practical limits upon the
quantity of material to be covered, but also to emphasize more
concisely and formally articulated statements of ethical and
other evaluative principles. These groups have not been limited to governing bodies of the entire religious denomination
(such as general assemblies and conventions). The collection
includes official resolutions and pronouncements of boards,
agencies, and councils within the denominational groups.

[7]For such a study, see Wilson Yates, *American Protestant-
ism and Birth Control: An Examination of Shifts with a Major
Religious Value Orientation* (unpublished Ph.D. dissertation,
Harvard University, 1968).

[8]The Federal Council of Churches (U.S.A.), "Excerpts from
Statement by Committee on Marriage and Home, 1931," in "A Compendium of Statements," collected by Richard M. Fagley (mimeographed, 1960), pp. 48-51.

"Responsible Parenthood and the Population Problem; Report of a Special Ecumenical Study Group," *Eugenics Quarterly*, VI, No. 4 (December, 1959), pp. 219-24.

Rabbi Ben Zion Bokser, "Statement on Birth Control." Final Draft Approved by The Committee on Jewish Law and Standards, (unpublished manuscript, January 31, 1961).

General Board of The National Council of the Churches of Christ in the U.S.A., "Responsible Parenthood," February 23, 1961 (pamphlet).

Pope Paul VI, "*Humanae Vitae*, 'On Human Life,'" in *The Catholic Case for Contraception*, ed. by Daniel Callahan (New York: The Macmillan Company, 1969), pp. 212-36.

The United Methodist Church, Board of Christian Social Concerns, "Population Resolutions," (pamphlet including resolutions on "Population Crisis" and "Responsible Parenthood" adopted October 6-9, 1969).

[9]Rabbi Ben Zion Bokser, "Statement on Birth Control," p. 3.

[10]The Federal Council of Churches (U.S.A.)--"Excerpts from Statement by Committee on Marriage and Home, 1931," p. 50.

[11]*Ibid.*

[12]Rabbi Ben Zion Bokser, "Statement on Birth Control," p. 1.

[13]Resolution on Responsible Parenthood of the General Conference of The Evangelical United Brethren Church, 1962, from an unpublished manuscript on file in the library of Planned Parenthood-World Population in New York, p. 1.

[14]Council for Christian Social Action (U.C.C.), "Responsible Parenthood and the Population Problem," adopted January, 1960, in "Compendium of Statements," pp. 39-40.

[15]Augustana Evangelical Lutheran Church, "Responsible Parenthood," adopted 1954, in "Compendium of Statements," pp. 31-32.

[16]Pope Paul, "*Humanae Vitae*," p. 225.

[17]Reformed Church in America, General Synod, "Divorce, Remarriage, and Planned Parenthood," (pamphlet dated June, 1962), p. 15.

[18]The United Methodist Church, Board of Christian Social Concerns, "Population Resolutions," resolution on "Responsible Parenthood." (italics added)

[19]Biserica Ortodoxa Romania (Jan.-Feb., 1967) cited in "Birth Control: Some Recent Orthodox Statements," *Eastern Churches Review*, II (1969), p. 69.

[20]Archbishop Michael, Greek Archdiocese of North and South America, 1956, in "Compendium of Statements," p. 43.

[21]Pius XI, *Casti Connubii*, translated in "Minority Papal Commission Report," in *The Catholic Case for Contraception*, p. 176.

[22]John T. Noonan, Jr., *The Church and Contraception: The Issues at Stake* (New York: Paulist Press, 1967), p. 2.

[23]*Ibid.*, pp. 2-3.

[24]"The Constitution of the Church in the Modern World," text in Noonan, *The Church and Contraception*, p. 53.

[25]Paul VI, *"Humanae Vitae,"* p. 220.

[26]"Majority Papal Commission Report," text in *The Catholic Case Against Contraception*, p. 159.

[27]Paul VI, *"Humanae Vitae,"* p. 220.

[28]"The Constitution of the Church in the Modern World," p. 54.

[29]"Majority Papal Commission Report," p. 155.

[30]Rabbi Ben Zion Bokser, "Statement on Birth Control," p. 1.

[31]Central Conference of American Rabbis, "Planned Parenthood and Overpopulation," from text on file in the library of Planned Parenthood-World Population, New York.

[32]*The Lambeth Conference: 1958* (London: S.P.C.K. and Seabury Press, 1958), p. 1-22. For other examples see The Protestant Episcopal Church, General Convention statement, "Christian Marriage and Population Control," 1961, the text of which is on file at the Planned Parenthood World Population library, New York; the statement which appeared in *Watch Tower*, the official journal of the Jehovah's Witnesses, March 1, 1951, p. 159, the text of which is also on file at the Planned Parenthood-World Population library; and The Federal Council of Churches (U.S.A.), "Excerpts from Statement by Committee on Marriage and Home, 1931," p. 48.

[33]Presbyterian Church in the U.S., "Action of the General Assembly, May, 1960," p. 36. See also "United Lutheran Church Statement," adopted October 16, 1956, text of which is on file at the Planned Parenthood-World Population library, New York.

[34]Pius XI, *Casti Connubii*, translated in "Minority Papal Commission Report," p. 176.

[35]Paul VI, *"Humanae Vitae,"* p. 224.

[36]"Statement by Rabbinical Alliance of America, 1958"; text is on file at the Planned Parenthood-World Population library, New York.

[37]Evangelical and Reformed Church, "Action of General Council, February, 1960," in "Compendium of Statements," p. 38.

[38]Reformed Church in America, General Synod, "Divorce, Remarriage, and Planned Parenthood," p. 15.

[39]The Protestant Episcopal Church, "Christian Marriage and Population Control," p. 19.

[40]Presbyterian Church in the U.S., "Action of the General Assembly," p. 36. Also see as examples, "Birth Control, Parenthood and Population," (from the Bishops Quadrennial Message, A.M.E. Zion Church, no date) text on file at the Planned Parenthood-World Population library, New York; *The Lambeth Conference: 1958*, p. 1:57; and The United Methodist Church, Board of Christian Social Concerns, "Population Resolutions," resolution on "Population Crisis."

[41]Rabbi Ben Zion Bokser, "Statement on Birth Control," pp. 1-2.

[42]Paul VI, *"Humanae Vitae,"* p. 213.

[43]John XXIII, *Mater et Magistra*, translated in "Minority Papal Commission Report," p. 178.

[44]See "United Lutheran Church Statement."

[45]See Paul VI, *"Humanae Vitae,"* p. 213.

[46]See United Presbyterian Church in the U.S.A., "Resolution Adopted by the 171st General Assembly, May, 1959," in "Compendium of Statements," p. 42, for an example.

[47]Council for Christian Social Action (U.C.C.), "Responsible Parenthood and the Population Problem," p. 40. We interpret "aesthetic" here to mean personal taste rather than an "objective" aesthetic value.

[48]Evangelical and Reformed Church, "Action of General Council, February, 1960," p. 38. See also The Federal Council of Churches (U.S.A.), "Excerpts from Statement by Committee on Marriage and Home, 1931," p. 48.

[49]Florence R. Kluckhohn and F. L. Strodtbeck, *Variations in Value Orientations* (Evanston, Ill.: Row, Peterson, 1961).

CHAPTER VII

AN EMPIRICAL STUDY OF PHYSICIAN DECISION-MAKING

INTRODUCTION

In Part I of this study we made many theoretical distinctions pertaining to the relations of values to the scientific and technological processes. In this and the following chapter we shall attempt to illustrate the interaction of evaluative and technological factors in the making of specific technical decisions. We have chosen to examine some of the decisions made by the physician as a concrete example of the significance of the value factor in technological decision-making. The physician's role, one of the most crucial and highly-respected in our society, is particularly fascinating. The physician is usually thought of as a great humanitarian servant. From the time of Hippocrates it has been recognized that medicine is an art, depending as it does upon the skill, technique, whims, and instincts of the performer. But first, and foremost, the modern physician is a highly trained applied scientist, a scientist who must apply his vast technical knowledge to the solving of very complex and critical human problems. In the practice of clinical medicine thousands of decisions are made daily in which values interact with technology.

In Chapter V we found that religion has been recognized as a major factor in the decisions physicians make about birth control. The Spivack study, however, was content to use a very crude indicator, religious affiliation, as the measure of this relationship. Religious affiliation, particularly when it is at the gross level of Catholic vs. non-Catholic, often can be far removed from the significant system of belief and value which is brought to bear on the decision-making process. The "cultural value complex," and particularly the moral component of the complex would seem to be a much more sensitive predictor of decision-making behavior. It is related to and partially dependent upon one's religious affiliation, to be sure, but it is also the product of the other significant groups and

persons in one's life. The cultural value complex also reflects the vast differences that are found within the various
religious denominations.

This chapter reports a study of 245 physicians. It was
designed to illustrate the importance of the cultural value
complex in physician decision-making and to test the following
hypotheses about this decision-making:

1. That the physician's moral judgments about birth
   control partially determine his beliefs about the
   non-moral facts. (Type IIc and IId inputs using
   the scheme devised in Chapter IV.)

2. That moral judgments are a major factor in determining the way physicians treat their patients
   regarding birth control. (Type III).

3. That the cultural value complex as measured by
   the cultural value scales is a better indicator
   of physician behavior than is his religious
   affiliation (cultural vs. social subsystem).

4. That physicians' evaluation and behavior regarding birth control have changed over a
   thirteen-year period from 1957 to 1970. (Type
   IIb).

We shall also seek answers to specific questions which
grow out of our previous discussion. Among these are:

1. What is the relationship between the moral and
   the hedonistic components in the cultural value
   complex?

2. What is the relationship between the moral and
   orientational components in the cultural value
   complex?

3. What is the relationship among the various
   moral factors in the cultural value complex?

In the next chapter we shall take a more intimate look at
the decision-making process reporting a case study of a community health system which included interviews with physicians and
their patients.

A. PREPARATION OF THE INSTRUMENT

The first method chosen to test these hypotheses and answer these questions was a survey questionnaire to be administered to a diverse sample of physicians who were either general

practitioners or obstetrician-gynecologists. It was decided
that a series of scales would be created reflecting the various
factors in the decision-making process. The construction of
the instrument took place in several stages. At first we were
working with a very simple model. A preliminary test instrument was written which contained basically two scales, one designed to measure moral judgments about oral contraception and
the other to measure beliefs about the non-evaluative scientific (pharmacological) facts. The original design was to examine
the relationship between these two factors. It can now be seen
in retrospect that we were dealing primarily within the scientific stage (Stage II). We were attempting to measure the extent to which moral judgments biased the reading of scientific
data.

This preliminary instrument was administered to 52 obstetricians by mail and personal interview in December, 1968. The
population for this phase consisted of the obstetricians in a
large Eastern city and two suburban mid-western towns.[1] The
results of this study indicated that a larger, more comprehensive investigation would be worthwhile. Work with that preliminary instrument and discussion with the physicians in the
study provided insights which have led to the distinctions made
in the later phases of this work.

Using the questions from the preliminary test, the final
instrument was constructed on the basis of the analysis of
church statements on birth control and family planning which we
have presented in Chapter VI. For each of the factors isolated
a scale was constructed consisting of approximately five items.
The questions consisted of Likert-type items and an additional
group of multiple choice items which could be scored in a manner similar to the Likert items.[2] The items for the construction of the scales were taken from or patterned after statements in the church position papers which we analyzed.

Three groups of scales were constructed. For the individual items in each scale, see Appendix II. The scales were:

A. Cultural Value Complex Scales

   1. Personal pleasure
   2. Ethical obligations related to population growth
   3. Ethical obligations related to the ends of marriage
   4. Ethical obligations related to sexual promiscuity

     5. Ethical obligations related to the "natural"
     6. General ethical obligations
     7. Value-orientations

B. Technical Scales

     1. Safety
     2. Effectiveness
     3. Demographic Facts

C. Application Scale (decisions made in clinical practice).

In order to test for changes which have taken place in physician attitudes in the last thirteen years, we repeated two of the items from the Spivack study of 1957. These dealt with the action of the physician when conducting a premarital (item 51) or a postpartum (item 55) examination when the patient did not bring up the subject of birth control. In the preliminary study these items were repeated exactly as in the Spivack study, but our pre-tests indicated that such shifts had taken place in the direction of initiation of birth control discussion that the overwhelming number of our physicians fell into Spivack's extreme category. (A full discussion of this shift will be presented below.) For this reason we increased the number of possible responses permitting a finer differentiation of practice in these situations. While this decreased the comparative value of the final instrument, it increased the sensitivity and differentiation.

The instrument also contained standard background items including religion, parents' religion, and the religious affiliation of the physician's medical school, and of his hospital. The completed instrument consisted of sixty-six items with a total of seventy-three responses due to some multiple response items. The completed instrument together with the covering explanatory letter are presented in Appendix I. In Appendix II a rearrangement of the items is presented showing the scales into which they were divided.

B. THE SAMPLE

In the selection of the sample for this study we were guided by several factors. First we wanted a wide distribution throughout the United States. We also wanted to include

physicians who were involved in birth control decision-making,
but exclude those who were not. It is important to note that
none of the hypotheses we were testing makes any claims about
the physician population in general. We are interested in the
relation of the various factors to one another *for an individual physician.* Nowhere will we claim that "physicians in general in the United States believe" this or that. This is important because we anticipated that in addition to having to
sample particular geographical areas we would have substantial
losses in the sample through non-returns. Thus we cannot even
make general descriptive statements about the physicians' views
in any one of the cities or counties in our sample.

1. *Sample Points.*

One of our objectives was to compare our findings with
those of Spivack. In order to facilitate this we decided to
duplicate his sample areas with certain modifications. Spivack
selected as his sample points six communities or clusters of
communities distributed throughout the United States with the
exception that no southern communities were included. His criteria for selection were:

> the rural-urban character of the population
> the educational level of the population
> the average family income of the population
> the proportion of Catholics in the population.[3]

On the basis of his criteria he selected three pairs of
sampling points, cities, towns, and rural areas, with each pair
having, insofar as possible, matched social and economic characteristics but varying in the proportion of Catholics. Some
of the demographic characteristics of the areas are shown in
Table 3. Space does not permit a full description of the characteristics of the areas. This is available in the description
of the study design for Spivack's study.[4]

We wanted to expand the sampling points for two reasons.
Since we were mailing a questionnaire while Spivack conducted
direct interviews, we were aware that our percentage return
would be smaller. Also, as we noted, there were no southern
sampling points. We decided to add a group of contiguous

TABLE 3

DEMOGRAPHIC DATA ON SAMPLE AREAS[1]

	Population 1950[2]	Population 1960	Percent Catholic[3]	Percent Urban	Median Age	Median School Years Completed	Median Family Income	Percent Women in Labor Force	Percent Professional in Labor Force
Low Catholic City	375,000	372,676	10.4	100	36.7	12.0	6335	40.2	51.3
High Catholic City	330,000	318,611	40.8	100	34.4	10.1	6361	42.4	41.3
Low Catholic Towns	135,000	176,008	22.6	41.8	33.4	10.3	6481	31.5	43.3
High Catholic Towns	140,000	158,093	40.9	58.2	31.4	11.2	5774	35.8	39.1
Low Catholic Rural	110,000	111,135	5.0	44.5	32.1	10.0	4652	30.5	33.8
High Catholic Rural	215,000	234,313	38.0	41.5	27.7	9.2	4927	31.9	30.4
Southern City		627,525	75.1	100	30.2	9.0	4807	35.4	44.4
Southern Town and Rural		733,393	78.7	38.3	22.9	7.3	3639	24.1	30.1

[1]Data except where indicated are taken from the 1960 census.

[2]Source: Cornish, *Doctors and Family Planning*, p. 77.

[3]Source: *Churches and Church Membership in the United States: An Enumeration and Analysis by Counties, States and Regions, Series C. Denominational Statistics by States and Counties* (New York: Bureau of Survey Research, National Council of Churches, 1957).

counties in a southern state which included city, town, and
rural characteristics and areas ranging from high Catholic to
virtually none. We knew that this area had fewer physicians
per capita and had reason to anticipate a smaller percentage
return. Therefore, this area was designed with a larger population than the other areas.

2. *Sample Selection.*

The sampling of the physicians within these areas was
based on a desire to reach those physicians who had relevant
patient contact in the area of contraception. Following Spivack, we included all physicians who indicate that their primary or secondary specialty is obstetrics and/or gynecology in
the twenty-fifth edition of the American Medical Directory.[5]
We also wanted to reach general practitioners. We included those physicians who indicated their primary area of practice was general practice, as a second sample group.[6] The numbers in the sample from the different sample points are shown
in Table 4. A questionnaire with postage-paid return envelope
was mailed to each physician in the sample during July, 1970.

TABLE 4

ORIGINAL SAMPLE AND NUMBER OF RESPONDENTS--BY AREA

Area	Original Sample	Respondents Respondents	Percent Return
Low Catholic City	159	52	33
High Catholic City	128	35	27
Low Catholic Towns	79	22	28
High Catholic Towns	77	22	29
Low Catholic Rural	39	15	38
High Catholic Rural	68	18	26
Southern City	174	44	25
Southern Town and Rural	173	37	21
TOTAL	897	245	27.3

A copy of the cover letter sent with each questionnaire is reproduced as Appendix III. A follow-up reminder letter was sent
to the non-respondents in High Catholic City five weeks after
the original mailing as a test of the utility of such a letter.
One additional response was received. No further follow-up
letters were sent.

3. *Non-respondents*.

In an empirical study of elites, the problem of non-
respondents is often a major one. In our case of the 897 in
the sample, 245 (27.3%) replied to our questionnaire with responses complete enough for incorporation into the analysis.[7]
This compares favorably with Guttmacher's 21.9% return for his
questionnaire on birth control mailed to physicians,[8] but does
not approach the 78% completion rate achieved by Spivack using
professional interviewers.[9]

The data in the American Medical Directory from which the
names were taken was supposed to be updated to August, 1969.
Thus it was eleven months out of date when the instrument was
mailed in July, 1970. Spivack, by sending interviewers to the
physicians' offices, was able to determine that ten percent of
his sample was unavailable or ineligible because the physicians
were no longer in active service, had left private practice, or
were no longer in the relevant fields. An additional twelve
percent refused to be interviewed. We are not able to determine the reason for lack of response to our questionnaire. We
are able, however, to say something about their characteristics. The non-respondents tended to be older than those who
responded. Twenty percent of those born before 1906 responded,
thirty-five percent of those born after 1925. The specialists
in obstetrics-gynecology were more likely to respond (thirty-
five percent compared to twenty-two percent for the general
practitioners group). We do not have a record of the religious
affiliation of the non-respondents although there is reason to
suppose that Catholics were less likely to respond. Comparing
the high Catholic and low Catholic areas, the low Catholic
sampling points had a thirty-one percent response while the
high Catholic sampling points had a twenty-seven percent

response. The southern area, which was also high Catholic, had a twenty-two percent response. Spivack does not reveal how he determined the religious affiliation of his refusers, but he reports that eleven percent of the non-Catholics available and eligible refused while twenty percent of the Catholics did. We anticipated such a difference but were also aware that we were drawing about half of our sample from high Catholic areas. Since Catholics are under-represented in the physician population, it is impossible to estimate exactly how our sample compares with the physician population in the areas we are studying. Of our respondents, 30.6% were Catholic, almost certainly reflecting the influence of the high Catholic areas in our sample. It is important to remember that we will make no claims for the physician population as a whole in our study.

C. DATA ANALYSIS

With each scale consisting of approximately five items, the scale score was calculated by taking the mean, following data recoding of certain items.[10] Combined scales were also calculated for the moral and the technical dimensions. These we shall refer to as the "morality" and "technical" scales respectively. The morality scales consisted of those items which contained either direct reference to "morally right," some other moral language, or the characteristics identified in Chapter III as the moral component of objectively legitimated evaluation. The technical scale was made up of those items with characteristics described in Chapter II as (non-evaluative) cognitive symbolization. We were able to program the computer to void any scale which had more than two items blank. In fact, very few blanks were present in the data. For the combined scales, a blank (void) scale score was recorded when more than four items were blank.[11]

Each scale score should be interpreted as meaning that the higher the scale score the more favorable the attitude toward oral contraception on the dimension of the scale. For instance, on the promiscuity scale, the higher the scale score, the less likely the respondent would be to object to oral contraception on the grounds that it would increase promiscuity.

On the natural morality scale, the higher the score, the less
likely the respondent would be to object to oral contraception
on the grounds that it is a violation of a moral requirement
that birth control should be limited to natural means. On the
safety scale, the higher the score, the safer the pill is
thought to be. On the application scale, the higher the score,
the more likely the physician would be to perform an act which
would lead to the use of oral contraception (such as bring up
the subject of birth control or prescribe oral contraception
under specified conditions). All data processing was done on
an IBM 7094 computer using the Data-Text system of data analysis. [12]

1. *The Cultural Value Complex.*

   We shall first discuss the responses on items dealing with
ethical and other evaluation dimensions. As stated above, we
originally developed seven evaluative dimensions, five of which
were specifically ethical. These ethical dimensions were related to (1) population growth, (2) the ends of marriage, (3)
sexual promiscuity, and (4) the "natural." In addition, four
very general morality items were grouped together as a "general
morality" scale. The questions grouped according to these
scales are reproduced in Appendix II. Also reproduced there
are the item-to-scale correlations showing the relation of each
item to the scale in which it is classified. We have also provided a record of the highest item-to-scale correlation for an
item not in the scale under consideration. It can be seen that
the item-to-scale correlations are high, ranging from .823
(item 23 which is in the promiscuity scale) to a low of .582
(item 32 which is in the population morality scale). The co-
hesiveness of the scales can be seen by the fact that there is
no single item which is not in a scale which has an item-to-
scale correlation for the scale under consideration as high as
any item listed in the scale. [13] Only rarely would it even be
the case that an item not in a given scale had an item-to-item
correlation with any item in the scale as high as any of the
item-to-item correlations for any of the items in the scale.

a. *The Ethical Dimensions*. Table 5 shows the inter-scale
correlation coefficient for all the scales we have developed.
As would be expected, all of the scales dealing with ethical
evaluation of oral contraception are highly intercorrelated.
That is to say, those who thought that oral contraception was
ethically unacceptable with regard to promiscuity also found it
ethically unacceptable with regard to the responsibilities of
marriage, found it in violation of ethical obligations regarding what is "natural," and did not believe demographic considerations to offer ethical claims supporting their use. It is
clear that ethical claims related to population were more
closely related to the ethical claims of responsible parenthood
than they were to the dimensions of promiscuity and the "natural." The issues in the "responsible parenthood" or "ends of
marriage" scale are directly related to the number of offspring
one has. The pro-contraception ethical claim is that one has a
responsibility as a parent to educate and care for offspring
requiring a limit to the number of children one has. The anti-
contraception claim is that one of the ends, the primary or
even the only end of marriage, is the production of offspring.
It is thus quite reasonable that the subscales dealing with the
ends of marriage and population are more closely related. In
Appendix V it can be seen that in the factor analysis these two
dimensions clustered together into what we have called the
"population and family-size factor."

While it was not our primary objective to investigate the
individual responses to items, many of them are inherently interesting. The response of a few are presented in Table 6. In
interpreting these, the restrictions on the representativeness
of our sample must be kept in mind.

b. *The Pleasure Scale*. While the ethical scales of the
cultural value complex reflected substantial homogeneity when
analyzed by examination of the correlation coefficients and
factor analysis, the "pleasure" scale gave a quite different
picture. These items seemed much more closely related to items
dealing with ethical or other types of propositions than with
other items from the pleasure scale. It would have been plausible for respondents to claim that oral contraception "avoids

TABLE 5

INTER-SCALE CORRELATION COEFFICIENTS

	Morality Scale	General	Promiscuity	Natural	Population Morality	Ends of Marriage	Technical	Safety	Effect-iveness	Population Facts	Pleasure	Applica-tion
Morality Scale	1.000	.795**	.802**	.799**	.630**	.824**	.624**	.525**	.183**	.480**	.610**	.773**
General Morality	.795**	1.000	.602**	.688**	.291**	.590**	.511**	.472**	.087	.361**	.488**	.716**
Promiscuity	.802**	.602**	1.000	.560**	.281**	.568**	.437**	.359**	.199**	.308**	.386**	.688**
Natural Morality	.799**	.688**	.560**	1.000	.316**	.604**	.521**	.468**	.124	.362**	.494**	.643**
Population Morality	.630**	.291**	.281**	.316**	1.000	.504**	.431**	.296**	.119	.457**	.428**	.376**
Ends of Marriage	.824**	.590**	.568**	.604**	.504**	1.000	.529**	.476**	.176*	.338**	.592**	.591**
Pleasure Scale	.610**	.488**	.386**	.494**	.428**	.592**	.526**	.483**	.156*	.353**	1.000	.466**
Technical Scale	.624**	.511**	.437**	.521**	.431**	.529**	1.000	.844**	.551**	.605**	.526**	.528**
Safety	.526**	.472**	.359**	.468**	.296**	.476**	.844**	1.000	.259**	.234**	.483**	.428**
Effectiveness	.183**	.087	.199**	.124	.119	.176**	.551**	.259**	1.000	.097	.156*	.228**
Population Facts	.480**	.361**	.308**	.362**	.457**	.338**	.605**	.234**	.097	1.000	.353**	.383**
Application Scale	.773**	.716**	.688**	.643**	.376**	.591**	.528**	.428**	.228**	.383**	.466**	1.000

*$p < .05$ **$p < .01$

TABLE 6

RESPONSES TO SELECTED MORALITY SCALE ITEMS
(blanks omitted from the percentages)

	Disagree strongly	Disagree	Disagree slightly	Agree slightly	Agree	Agree strongly
The increased use of birth control pills by unmarried girls indicates a decline in American morality.	28 (12%)	77 (33%)	12 (5%)	37 (16%)	47 (20%)	33 (14%)
One of the ends of marriage is the production of offspring. Those who seek to avoid offspring without medical reason may be acting selfishly.	72 (30%)	78 (33%)	12 (5%)	24 (10%)	34 (14%)	17 (7%)
The interests of one's family override any obligations to society in determining family size.	48 (20%)	68 (29%)	33 (14%)	24 (10%)	35 (15%)	26 (11%)
There is something unjust about a couple with three children and substantial family income choosing to have another child.	77 (33%)	81 (34%)	37 (16%)	21 (9%)	13 (6%)	6 (3%)
To be fair to the other children a couple has a moral obligation to try to limit pregnancies by a means as reliable as the pill.	12 (5%)	39 (16%)	21 (9%)	39 (16%)	85 (36%)	40 (17%)
It is not morally justifiable for any outside agency to infringe on a couple's right to have children.	36 (15%)	52 (22%)	24 (10%)	27 (11%)	44 (19%)	51 (22%)
It would be desirable from a moral point of view to have a reliable contraceptive means which was natural rather than artificial.	21 (9%)	33 (14%)	19 (8%)	48 (21%)	63 (27%)	46 (20%)
It is morally preferable to limit birth control to natural means such as abstinence and rhythm.	113 (48%)	61 (26%)	19 (8%)	11 (5%)	18 (8%)	13 (6%)
Access to hormonal steroids for contraception should be carefully controlled in order to minimize promiscuity.	69 (30%)	52 (23%)	30 (13%)	30 (13%)	31 (14%)	18 (8%)

unpleasantness of other methods" (item 3), but that it was
still immoral. It would have been plausible to claim that the
pill was safe (measured by the safety scale), but still that
"there is something unpleasant about having to take a pill
daily as a means of conception control" (item 38). This did
not seem to be the usual case, however. Finding the pill pleasurable was closely linked to finding it moral (r=.610, p <
.01). This does not necessarily mean that moral judgments are
nothing more than judgments about individual pleasure. It
could be that displeasure associated with the pill arises from
the judgment that it is immoral or it could be that feelings of
pleasure are, in some cases, used as the data for making moral
judgments. Finding the pill pleasurable is also linked to
finding it safe (r=.483, p < .01). Again, this may mean nothing more than that displeasure is seen as arising out of use of
the pill because it is dangerous.

The report of the factor analysis presented in Appendix V
reveals that two of the pleasure items were more closely related to the safety dimensions (items 35 and 38). Two of the
items were more closely related to the evaluative dimensions
(items 30 and 46). One of the items showed about equal relation to the safety and evaluative elements (item 18). The
highly complex interaction between the scales we are studying
does not permit a causal analysis under the present design.
However, when we discuss the interaction between the morality
and technical scales, we shall offer some argument relating to
the causal relationship in that interaction.

c. *The Orientational Values*. In addition to the ethical
and hedonistic dimensions we included a total of nine items
which attempted to operationalize the orientational values of
Kluckhohn and Strodtbeck[14] which we presented in Chapter III.
Some of the responses are shown in Table 7. A full measure
of the five orientational values would have required many more
items than we could include in the present study. Our observations here are, thus, very tentative and preliminary.

We were working with five different orientational values
(man/nature, time, good/evil, activity, and relation as described in Chapter III). There was no theoretical reason for

TABLE 7

SELECTED RESPONSES TO ORIENTATIONAL VALUE ITEMS

(blanks omitted from the percentage)

Item	Disagree strongly	Disagree	Disagree slightly	Agree slightly	Agree	Agree strongly
The physician's role is to become a part of our great technology in which man is subduing nature.	39 (17%)	57 (25%)	18 (8%)	42 (18%)	51 (22%)	22 (10%)
People do not have enough respect for time honored traditions these days. We should work hard to keep up those good things from the past.	27 (12%)	37 (16%)	26 (11%)	54 (23%)	64 (27%)	23 (10%)
I consider myself very much an individual. I would rather work by myself than with a team or for someone else.	18 (8%)	44 (19%)	22 (9%)	37 (16%)	55 (23%)	58 (25%)
When it comes right down to it, there is a basic tendency toward evil in most men.	47 (20%)	65 (28%)	29 (12%)	31 (13%)	38 (16%)	22 (9%)
What I care about most is accomplishing things; I like to see results and think they are worth working for.	2 (1%)	7 (3%)	15 (6%)	40 (17%)	101 (43%)	67 (29%)

them to be interrelated but Kluckhohn and Strodtbeck have
found patterns to be characteristic of cultural groups suggesting that there is some empirical basis for patterns of inter-
relations. We had anticipated that there might be analogous
characteristic orientational value patterns within a cultural
group such as physicians. We found preliminary evidence that
such patterns may exist, but the evidence weak. Factor 4 in
our factor analysis (Appendix V) incorporates six of the nine
orientational value items (items 10, 22, 31, 19, 16, and 34).
This suggests that a common factor relates to physicians' attitudes about the relation between man and nature, orientation
toward the present, individuality, and activity. Examination
of the inter-item correlation matrix for these items suggests
that inter-relations do exist among these items, but that the
relationships as measured are very weak. It would be sheer
speculation to comment any further on the basis of the evidence
at hand. We plan further work testing the relation of orientational values to medical decision-making in the future.

The relationship of the orientational value items to the
morality items is interesting. Looking first at the overall
morality scale we find that no single orientational item corre-
lates as highly as .3. The dimension of the relationship between man and nature cannot be shown to be significantly related to the morality scale.[15] The symmetric lambda measure of
association is 0.080. Likewise, no significant relationship
was found between the time orientation and the morality scale.
In this case the symmetric lambda measure of association was
0.092.

Even more interesting is the lack of a demonstrable relationship between the man/nature orientation and the subscale
of the morality scale which measures the claim that oral contraception is morally wrong because it is unnatural. This suggests that the discussion about the "naturalness" of contraception has become a separate, autonomous argument independent of
the man/nature orientation more generally conceived.

2. *The Relation of Moral and Other Evaluative Judgments to Beliefs about Technical Facts.*

One of the primary objectives of our study was to investigate the relationship of value judgments related to oral contraception and beliefs about the non-evaluative facts. In Chapter IV we developed a model of decision-making in which these two elements were considered the primary factors in decision-making. Evaluative propositions were seen as the major premise and non-evaluative, cognitive propositions were the minor premise of a syllogism. But we also argued that there were complications in this model. Statements of non-evaluative facts may be selected in such a way that they are value-loaded: i.e., they may combine with evaluations about which there is common agreement to lead necessarily to decisions about actions. Statements about non-evaluative facts may also be biased by particular interests. Within the scientific stage two of the value factors we identified were choices related to method and other selections (Type IId) and bias and distortion (Type IIc). Type IId includes selection from among available data those which are "worth" considering and reporting.

One or both of these value factors appear to have been present in the responses in our study of physicians. One of the most important findings in this study has been the relationship of moral judgments to beliefs about technical facts. As described above, we created scales dealing with moral judgments and beliefs about technical facts. We have called these the morality and technical scales respectively. As shown in Table 5, the correlation coefficient is .624 (p < .01). The correlations between the morality scale and the technical subscales ranged from .183 to .526, all significant. This means that to a great extent the more moral the pill was judged, the more safe and effective it was thought to be and the more rapidly population was thought to be growing and resources vanishing.

While this shows a remarkable relationship between statements about morality and statements about non-evaluative facts, it does not tell us exactly what the basis of the relation is. Further analyzing the data and the content of the questions

gives some hints about how the relation is brought about. One
of the first questions which arises is that of directionality.
It is logically possible, though it seems unlikely, that a physician maintains that oral contraception is immoral, but only
because it is physically dangerous. In response to the statement, "I would have to classify oral contraceptive therapy as a
morally questionable 'artificial' means of limiting conception"
(item 27), a physician could respond, although on the surface
it seems unlikely, "Yes, I agree, but only because the pill is
dangerous and using a dangerous drug is immoral." If any judgment is to be made about directionality, we have to know if
beliefs about technical facts are being read into presumably
moral judgments in this way. It should be made clear that this
influence should only be present for the group that believes
oral contraception to be technically unsafe or ineffective, but
otherwise morally acceptable. For the other three possible
combinations (safe and otherwise moral, safe but otherwise immoral, and unsafe and otherwise immoral) this influence should
not measurably change the relationship of morality to technical
scales.

In the pre-test, we made the following statistical calcu-
lation. We noted that some of the items in the morality scale
could, theoretically, have beliefs about technical facts incorporated as illustrated above. On the other hand, there were
other morality scale items where this seems logically impossible. For instance, item 35 ("the possibility that the pill
might lead to increased promiscuity raises moral questions
about its widespread availability") would appear to be independent of whether the pill is safe or dangerous. Classifying
the morality scale items on this basis, we found eleven items
of the type which were, in content, independent of the technical data and ten items which theoretically could be influenced
by the position that the pill is immoral, but only because it
is unsafe. From this we generated two subscales. For want of
a better term, we called the first the "pure morality scale"
and the second the "impure morality scale." We then set about
to correlate the two subscales to the technical scales. If
the directionality of the correlation was really that of

technical facts being incorporated into moral judgments, we
would expect the impure morality scale to correlate highly
with the technical scale and the pure morality scale to be unrelated. However, the results were dramatic. The impure morality scale, which we would expect to be the only one correlated to the technical scale if this rather circuitous moral
logic were operating, correlated with r=.516. The pure morality scale which should be unrelated if this logic is operating
showed a correlation of r=.520. This is strong evidence that
those reading the morality scale items were reading them in a
straightforward way and not mentally arguing that the pill is
immoral, but only because it is dangerous. Examination of the
item-to-scale correlations between the morality scale items and
the technical scale confirms this conclusion. The items which
were "pure" tended to show about the same correlations as those
which were theoretically "impure."

From the interviews we conducted with physicians, we can
get some idea of how the interaction takes place. Picking up
the item in the questionnaire about whether there was evidence
the pill caused cancer and whether the death rates from throm-
boembolism were higher among pill takers we asked the physicians we interviewed open-ended questions designed to elicit
how the physician would respond to such inquiries from a patient. For instance, we would ask, "Doctor, if your patient
asked you if the pill would cause cancer, how would you respond?" The differences were remarkable.

One physician, who could be identified as having serious
moral doubts about oral contraception on the basis of his questionnaire response and his subjective remarks, responded:

> Nothing has been proven. There are two opinions.
> One says we should worry; another says don't
> worry. There is definite controversy on this
> matter and if we are going to use the pill, we
> have to accept some risks.

In other interviews men would mention evidence of carcino-
genic changes in the cells of test animals given chemicals re-
sembling oral progesterones.

On the other hand, a physician thoroughly committed to the
morality of oral contraception replied:

No! I would tell them no. I don't think it
causes cancer. Maybe the pill will bring about
a tumor factor--so will pregnancy. I don't think
I'm making cancer in women. I can discuss it
scientifically.

Another physician responded:

No study has shown there is an association of
cancer with the pill. There might have been
benign tumors in rats, but that is absurd. Those
pills had natural progesterones.

These all seem to be cases where physicians are reporting
information reasonably accurately from the scientific literature, but the tone is very different. There is clearly a
selection of information considered important and different in
emphasis. These we called Type IId value factors in Chapter
IV. As long as questions are kept fairly general--of the kind
a layman might ask his physician--there are great opportunities
for value inputs even in reporting the technical information.
A physician *must* choose what he considers important to read and
to communicate to his patients. There is no way of avoiding
these value incorporating decisions.

Looking at the subscales (Table 5), it is apparent that
the morality scale was more closely related to the safety component than the effectiveness. Estimates of pregnancy rates
(item 50) correlated with the morality scale (r=.273, p < .01)
while estimates of how often the physician, assuming he and his
patient had no moral objections, would refuse to prescribe oral
contraceptives because of the risk of side effects correlated
with r=.380 (p < .01). Some of this difference can probably
be accounted for by the differences in the questions asked, but
even with this taken into account it appears that estimates of
safety are more vulnerable to these value inputs.

Looking at the subscales of the morality scale, items
dealing with the ends of marriage and the artificiality of oral
contraception appeared to be more closely related to the technical scale than did items dealing with promiscuity and population ethics. Again, this may be a result of the specific items
so no firm conclusion should be drawn.

The relationship of the pleasure scale to the technical
scale also shows a highly significant correlation (r=.526,

p < .01). The directionality in this case is much more ambiguous. We have already noted in the discussion of the factor
analysis that two of the pleasure scale items were treated by
respondents more like safety items. These were item 3 (Setting
aside questions of morality, the "pill" is one of the most convenient methods of birth control available and avoids much unpleasantness of other methods) and item 38 (There is something
unpleasant about having to take a pill daily as a means of contraception control). Another item (number 18) loaded about
equally on the factor for safety and the one which included the
items of the promiscuity, ends of marriage, and natural morality scales. It appears that personal pleasures and displea-
sures related to oral contraception are associated with both
moral judgments and judgments about non-evaluative facts. Additional study with more precise discrimination in the questions would be needed to analyze the pleasure dimension of the
cultural value complex more fully.

The relationship between orientational values and beliefs
about the technical facts were also examined. We anticipated
that the man/nature orientation and the time orientation might
show some relation. This was substantiated by the data, but
the relations are small. The statement, "The physician's role
is to become a part of our great technology in which man is
subduing nature," (item 10) was designed to measure the man
over nature dimension. Affirmation of this statement showed a
small, but significant positive correlation with the technical
scale ($r=.153$, $p < .05$). Those who thought the pill more safe
and effective, who thought population to be growing more rapidly and resources vanishing more rapidly, also tended to think
that the physician's role was to subdue nature. A correlation
($r=.194$, $p < .01$) was found between the technical scale and an
item (number 31) designed to measure the nature over man dimension ("The forces of nature are awe inspiring. The physician
best serves his function if he has respect for the complexity
of the human body and counts on nature to do its own healing").
The item designed to measure the good/evil orientation also
showed a significant correlation with the technical scale
($r=.153$, $p < .05$). The more the physician disagreed with the

notion that there is a basic tendency toward evil in most men
(item 25), the higher his score on the technical scale. None
of the other value orientation items could be shown to have a
significant relationship with the technical scale. Some responses to technical scale items are shown in Table 8.

3. *The Relation of Moral Judgments and Beliefs about Technical
   Facts to Decisions about Application.*

We have just illustrated the way in which values are related to beliefs about technical facts. These are examples of
the value inputs at the scientific stage (Types IIc and d). In
Chapter IV we also analyzed value inputs at the post-scientific
or application stage (Type III). The application scale in our
questionnaire consists of a series of ten items designed to
measure decisions physicians make in the course of their medical practice. They included questions about whether the physician would prescribe oral contraceptives under certain specified conditions and whether he would bring up the subject of
contraception under specified conditions. (See Appendix II for
the items in the scale.) In terms of the structure of decision-
making discussed in Chapter IV, the scientific stage includes
the filling in of the minor premise. Values are incorporated
here through bias and distortion (Type IIc) and selection
choices (Type IId). When we come to clinical decisions that a
physician must make about what to tell his patient or what to
prescribe, values must be incorporated much more directly.
Evaluative propositions are the major premise of the decision-
making logic. Some of the responses to items dealing with
clinical application are presented in Tables 9 and 10.

The physician shares with any applied scientist the dilemma of possessing competence in a particular functionally specific area and a commitment to minimize the value inputs into the
scientific process of handling information within that area
while at the same time being routinely expected to make decisions and recommendations which require a system of evaluation.
The decisions and recommendations will be the resultant of both
an evaluative symbol system and a (non-evaluative) scientific,
cognitive symbol system. We would expect that the decisions

TABLE 8

SELECTED RESPONSES TO TECHNICAL SCALE ITEMS
(blanks omitted from the percentages)

Item	Disagree strongly	Disagree	Disagree slightly	Agree slightly	Agree	Agree strongly
There is some evidence that oral contraceptives produce cancer.	86 (37%)	73 (31%)	24 (10%)	26 (11%)	16 (7%)	5 (2%)
Death rates from thromboembolic disease are substantially higher from women on the pill than for those of the same age not on the pill.	27 (12%)	71 (31%)	25 (11%)	53 (23%)	40 (17%)	12 (5%)
The population growth in the United States is one of the lowest for the developed countries of the world.	18 (8%)	74 (34%)	42 (19%)	29 (13%)	40 (18%)	9 (4%)
Skipping one pill near mid-cycle in the twenty-day cycle greatly increases the chance of conception.	33 (14%)	74 (32%)	35 (15%)	36 (16%)	42 (18%)	12 (5%)

TABLE 9

SELECTED RESPONSES TO APPLICATION SCALE ITEMS

Item	Fulfill the request	Explain other methods then fulfill request	Encourage other methods then fulfill request	Refer to another physician	Refer to clergyman	Refuse request
A 16 year old unmarried girl requesting oral contraceptives.	82 (37%)	18 (8%)	8 (4%)	1 (.4%)	17 (8%)	95 (43%)
A 26 year old unmarried girl requesting oral contraceptives.	172 (76%)	10 (4%)	7 (3%)	1 (.4%)	3 (1%)	32 (14%)
A Catholic patient who requests oral contraceptives.	184 (82%)	24 (11%)	2 (1%)	0	6 (3%)	9 (4%)

TABLE 10

SELECTED RESPONSES ON APPLICATION SCALE ITEMS

In a premarital examination, if the patient does not bring up the subject of contraception, how often do you?

	1970	1970[1] (excluding Southern)	1968[2]	1957[3]
always	97 (43%)	74 (47%)	—	—
very often	28 (12%)	15 (10%)	36 (69%)	22%
often	13 (6%)	7 (4%)	7 (13%)	11%
fairly often	12 (5%)	9 (6%)	—	—
occasionally	32 (14%)	22 (14%)	6 (12%)	20%
never	46 (20%)	29 (18%)	3 (6%)	47%

If your postpartum patients don't ask for advice on child-spacing, how often do you introduce the subject?

	1970	1970[1] (excluding Southern)	1968[2]	1967[3]
always	94 (44%)	66 (45%)	—	—
almost always	43 (20%)	28 (19%)	38 (73%)	27%
very often	10 (5%)	7 (5%)	—	—
often	13 (6%)	11 (7%)	—	—
sometimes	27 (12%)	17 (12%)	12 (23%)	23%
hardly ever	11 (5%)	8 (5%)	2 (4%)	50%
never	18 (8%)	9 (6%)	—	—

If a woman with three children, good health, and substantial family income expresses a desire for further children, how likely would you be to suggest to her that population growth is a factor to be considered in family planning?

certain	21 (9%)
very likely	13 (5%)
likely	30 (13%)
unlikely	73 (31%)
very unlikely	51 (21%)
certain not to	50 (21%)

---

[1]Excluding Southern sample points from our sample points makes our geographical areas identical to Spivack's 1957 study.

[2]Based on our pre-test results sampling one large Eastern city and two Mid-Western suburban towns.

[3]Cornish, *Doctors and Family Planning*, p. 40.

made about application of scientific knowledge would reflect
both of those elements.

This is exactly what we found with the particular set of
measures we made with our sample of physicians. Looking first
at the relation between the belief about technical facts (as
measured by the technical scale) and decisions made in clinical
practice (as measured by the application scale), we found a
correlation of .528 (p < .01). This is quite reasonable; the
safer the pill is, the more likely a physician is to follow
practices which would lead to its use. The more effective it
is, the more likely he is to follow those practices. In effect
safety, effectiveness, and demographic facts are "value-loaded."
We may presume safety, effectiveness, and, to some extent,
demographic conditions carry with them evaluations about which
there is some consensus.

We also found that there was a correlation of .773 (p <
.01) between the morality and the application scales. At
first, this might appear to be an undesirable state of affairs.
However, upon reflection, it should become evident that this
is not at all a "bad" situation. It does not mean physicians
are biased. Let us hope that actions taken by physicians,
scientists, and all human beings would, in some way, be related
to what they think to be right or wrong. Perhaps the last hint
of humanness has left *homo scienticus* when he can say, "Abortion is murder, but that doesn't bother me. I practice my
medicine in a value-free manner." The correlation between the
morality scale and the application scale indicates that these
physicians have not become practitioners according to the "engineering model" discussed in Chapter IV. They do not practice
their specialty with no questions asked.

The dilemma remains, however. The higher the correlation
between the professional's moral and other evaluative judgments
and his decisions in the application stage, the more his own
system of evaluation is being incorporated in the action. The
professional is in danger of the excesses of the clinical model
discussed in Chapter IV. The higher the correlation between
the evaluative system of the professional and the decisions
made, the more the lay actor's legitimate claims are jeopardized. He is entitled to have decisions about which he is the

primary subject made on the basis of a system of values which
are either his own or which, in the case where with due process
society has acted to impose the common interest, are those of
the society. There is a grave danger of generalization of expertise in which the professional is assumed to possess expertise in the system of evaluation as well as the technical facts
which are incorporated into the decision-making process. The
only way we know of by which this dilemma can be avoided is to
develop some system whereby there is reason to assume that the
professional's system of evaluation is compatible with that of
the lay actor who is directly involved. Depending upon the
societal conditions at a particular moment in history this will
be brought about by the adoption of the collegial or the contractual model of professional-lay relationships.

There is one further complicating problem. We already
have seen that beliefs about the non-evaluative facts are
closely related to evaluative judgments. That being the case,
even if it could be shown that there was a perfect correlation
between beliefs about the technical (non-evaluative) facts and
application, we could not be sure that the professional's evaluative system was not being incorporated indirectly. We appear
to have a system where application decisions are based both on
the technical and evaluative systems, while the technical system itself is dependent upon the evaluative system. Below we
shall complicate the picture even further when we discuss the
possibility of feedback loops indicating that the evaluative
system itself is dependent upon technical and application factors.

4. *Background Characteristics.*

In our discussion of an integrated model for decision-
making in Chapter II, we included the organic, psychological,
and social systems of the professional actor and, as part of
the social system, the professional actor's primary social
reference--the professional social system. That components
from these spheres influence decisions cannot be denied. They
become the secondary factors in the decision-making logic and
influence the primary factors as well. We have obtained for

each respondent his religious affiliation, parents' affiliation, sponsorship of his medical school, sponsorship of his
hospital, his age, sex, specialty, and geographical location.
We have cross-tabulated each of these background variables. We
have also cross-tabulated each with the scale scores. Since
most of the background scales are nominal (they cannot be arranged in an ordinal series) we have had to resort to cross-
tabulation rather than correlation. In order to do this, we
divided the scale scores into quartiles generating four groups
for each scale. The entire cross-tabulation series generated
255 contingency tables--a mass of data for which we cannot possibly report more than the highlights. (Note that that is an
instance of a Type IId value input.)

   a. *Parents' Religious Affiliation, Respondent's Religious
Affiliation, Medical School Sponsorship and Hospital Affiliation*. These four background variables constitute an interrelated set. We have hypothesized a model in which parents'
religious affiliation predicts respondent's religious affiliation, which in turn predicts medical school sponsorship and
hospital sponsorship. These four factors taken together might
be expected to partially determine both the cultural value complex and the beliefs about technical facts which are incorporated into the decision-making process. These in turn interact
to produce the decision.

   For parents and respondents, we provided alternatives of
Protestant, Catholic, Jewish, and Other. For Protestant and
Other, an opportunity was provided for the respondent to speci-
fy, but no analysis has been performed as yet on the subgroup-
ings. For the purposes of this analysis, two additional categories were generated: non-Catholic (some combination of more
than one of the non-Catholic categories) and Catholic plus non-
Catholic. These were used when parents had more than one religious affiliation. We were also able to calculate several regression equations. In order to do this, the nominal data were
dichotomized, for instance, into Catholic and non-Catholic.
The results of the cross-tabulations are shown in Table 11.
They are expressed with two terms--first, the probability of a
significant relationship in each of the cross-tabulations
based on the Chi Square Test (indicated by "p") and, second,

TABLE 11

RESULTS OF CROSS-TABULATION OF RELIGIOUS AFFILIATIONS

	Respondent's Religion	Medical School Affiliation	Hospital Affiliation	Morality Scale Quartiles	Technical Scale Quartiles	Application Scale Quartiles
Parents' Religion	$p < .001$ $V = .577$	$p = .079$ $V = .187$	$p < .001$ $V = .237$	$p < .001$ $V = .278$	$p = .009$ $V = .216$	$p < .001$ $V = .254$
Respondent's Religion		$p = .395$ $V = .163$	$p < .001$ $V = .232$	$p < .001$ $V = .291$	NS $V = .139$	$p < .001$ $V = .245$
Medical School Affiliation			$p < .001$ $V = .225$	$p = .226$ $V = .179$	$p = .126$ $V = .195$	$p = .230$ $V = .182$
Hospital Affiliation				$p = .328$ $V = .171$	NS $V = .095$	$p = .011$ $V = .229$

p = probability of significance of the Chi Square Test.

V = Cramer's V measure of association.

the Cramer V statistic, a measure of association with a range
of zero to one.

From this it can be seen that religion and parents' religion are the most closely associated with both the morality and
application scale quartiles. Those relationships are all significant with p < .001. The degree of association, however, is
not high. Cramer's V statistic is in the range of .24 to .29.
The association of parents' religion and respondent's religion
to the technical scale is even smaller. From our regression
equations we were able to calculate that parents' religion and
respondent's religion together accounted for twenty-three percent of the variance in the morality scale and only six percent
of the variance in the technical scale. All of this supports
the important conclusion that, while parents' religious affiliation and respondent's religious affiliation are the sociological variables which are the best predictors of the morality
scale scores, they are not particularly good predictors. The
correlation of religious affiliation (expressed as Catholic vs.
non-Catholic) with the decisions expressed in clinical practice (expressed as the application scale score) is .412. The
correlation of the moral evaluation of oral contraception (expressed in the morality scale) and clinical decisions is .773.
If one looks at religious affiliation rather than directly at
the moral judgments, he loses a great deal of precision.

On the cross-tabulation of the respondent's religion with
the morality scale scores divided into quartiles, ten percent
of the Catholics in the sample were in the fourth quartile
(i.e., ranking the respondents according to how moral they believed oral contraception to be, they were in the upper quarter). In contrast, fourteen percent of all of the Protestants
were in the lowest quartile.

To our surprise, no significant relationship could be
found between either parents' religious affiliation or respondent's religious affiliation and the affiliation of the medical
school the respondent attended. In turn, medical school affiliation was a poor predictor of morality, technical, and application scale scores. While parents' and respondent's religious
affiliations taken together account for 22.99 percent of the

variance in the morality scale score, adding medical school
affiliation raises this to only 23.04 percent. Apparently,
medical school is playing a very small role in determining the
morality scale. A similar conclusion can be reached for the
technical scale, the percent variance explained rising from
6.43 to 6.95 percent.

Sponsorship of the hospital of the respondent is more
closely associated with parents' religious affiliation (V =
.237) and respondent's religious affiliation (V = .232). While
hospital sponsorship cannot be shown to be significantly related to the morality scale or the technical scale, there is a
fairly low (V = .229) but significant (p = .011) relationship
with the clinical decisions measured by the application scale.

In summary, our conclusion is that parents' and respondent's religious affiliations are the best predictors of moral
judgments, beliefs about the non-evaluative facts, and clinical
decisions; they, nevertheless, are not particularly good predictors. By measuring directly the moral judgments (expressed
in the morality scale) and the beliefs about the non-evaluative
facts (expressed in the technical scale), we have a much better
predictor of clinical decisions (expressed as the application
scale).

b. *Geographical Area.* Compared with the sociological
variables which include religious affiliation as a dimension,
the other background variables (geographical area, medical
specialty, age, and sex) show even less of an association with
the moral judgments, beliefs about non-evaluative facts, and
clinical decisions measured by their respective scales (see
Table 12). The physicians in our sample were selected from
eight different geographical areas. It must be remembered that
geographical areas were selected on the basis of Catholicity of
the population. There is an expected association between geographical area and respondent's religion (V = .213) though it
is not significant due to the high number of degrees of freedom
in the cross-tabulation. Partially because of the religious
factor, geographical area was associated with the morality
scale (V = .200), technical scale (V = .234), and application
scale (V = .235) though none of these associations is significant.

TABLE 12

RESULTS OF CROSS-TABULATION OF OTHER BACKGROUND VARIABLES

	Sex	Specialty	Geographical Area	Morality Scale Quartiles	Technical Scale Quartiles	Application Scale Quartiles
Age	$p = .050$ $V = .201$	$p = .015$ $V = .187$	NS $V = .202$	NS $V = .111$	NS $V = .127$	$p = .011$ $V = .197$
Sex		$p = .125$ $V = .156$	NS $V = .113$	$p = .273$ $V = .130$	$p = .063$ $V = .183$	NS $V = .099$
Specialty			$p < .001$ $V = .309$	NS $V = .108$	NS $V = .115$	$p < .001$ $V = .204$
Geographical Area				NS $V = .200$	$p = .286$ $V = .234$	$p = .256$ $V = .235$

p = probability of significance of the Chi Square Test

V = Cramer's V measure of association

c. *Medical Specialty*. Our sample was made up of obstetrician-gynecologists and general practitioners. Medical specialty showed an association with geographical area (V = .309,
p < .001). While it could not be shown to be significantly
related to the morality and technical scales, it was to the
application scale (V = .204, p < .001).

d. *Age*. We pointed out in Chapter V that there have been
substantial differences in previous studies in the importance
of age as a variable. Our study showed weak associations with
the morality and technical scales (which were not significant)
and a significant association with the application scale (V =
.197, p = .011). Using ten-year age groups beginning with age
thirty-five, we found a slight tendency for younger men to look
with more favor on clinical decisions favoring oral contraception. Looking directly at the age factor's relation to the
application scale, the correlation was r=.249, p < .01.

e. *Sex*. The final variable to be considered is the sex of
the respondent. No significant relationships were found between sex and any of the scales in our study. It was found
that females were more likely to agree with the statement that
"Skipping one pill near mid-cycle in the twenty-day cycle
greatly increases the chance of conception" (r=.208, p < .01).
Other than that, sex appears to have been the least important
of the variables.

5. *Changes in Decision-Making over Time*.

Thus far we have spoken of the many ways values are incorporated into decision-making. In Chapter IV our cybernetic
model included the idea of feedback loops from the scientific
and post-scientific stages to values. It has often been assumed that changes in the state of scientific knowledge and
policies regarding the use of that knowledge have an input on
values. In order to examine changes in clinical decision-
making during the period of the last decade which has witnes-
sed major changes in contraceptive technology, we included in
our study two questions asked by Spivack in his 1957 study.
The results are summarized in Table 10. Since our sample included two additional sampling points (a Southern city and a

Southern town and rural area), we have also given the results
of our study with those geographical areas excluded.

We also asked these questions in our pre-test in 1968.
The sampling points for this phase were different (a large
Eastern city and two Mid-Western suburbs). We did not want to
pre-test in our final sample area. Therefore, those results
are not strictly comparable. In the pre-test, we asked the
Spivack questions with his response categories. Even though it
was a different population, the comparison between the 1957 and
1968 results is dramatic. In response to the questions, "In a
premarital examination, if the patient does not bring up the
subject of contraception, how often do you?" Spivack found only
twenty-two percent responded "very frequently." Forty-seven
percent said "never." In our pre-test sample with the same response choices (very frequently, often, occasionally, and
never), we found sixty-nine percent said "very frequently,"
while only six percent said "never."

We also duplicated a question in which we inquired about
how often the physician would introduce the subject of child
spacing if the patient did not solicit his advice. From the
response choices of "almost always," "sometimes," and "hardly
ever, never," Spivack found twenty-seven percent said "almost
always" and fifty percent said "hardly ever, never." In 1968
with our pre-test group, we found seventy-three percent said
"almost always" and four percent said "hardly ever, never."
Such dramatic shifts are very convincing evidence that change
has taken place even when we realize that we were dealing with
different samples.

Since over two-thirds of our responses were in one category on both questions, we decided to provide additional response choices in the final study where we were duplicating
Spivack's sample. We realized that this would decrease compar-
ability, but wanted to increase the discriminatory power of our
questions. Comparing our 1970 results with Spivack's from 1957
for the same populations (i.e., excluding the Southern sampling
points in our data), we found that forty-seven percent of the
physicians in 1970 would introduce the subject of contraception
in the pre-marital examination "always," and another ten percent "very often." This contrasts with the twenty-two percent

who picked the "very frequently" choice in 1957. While forty-seven percent said "never" in 1957, only eighteen percent did so in 1970. In response to the question of the postpartum exam, forty-five percent said "always." This contrasts to twenty-seven percent who said "almost always" in 1957. In 1970, five percent said "hardly ever" and six percent said "never" compared to fifty percent who said "hardly ever, never" in 1957. We find this to be dramatic evidence that there has been a major shift in the physician's conception of what is appropriate decision-making in medical practice in the thirteen-year period.

SUMMARY

This completes our report of a study of decision-making by 245 physicians regarding oral contraception. Our objective has not been to claim that American physicians or even physicians in the communities we studied have certain values and make particular decisions. Rather, our objective was to examine the interactions among various components in the decision-making process. We first examined the empirical measures of the cultural value complex. We found that among the ethical factors in the cultural value complex the dimensions relating to promiscuity, the ends of marriage, and the artificiality of contraception clustered together. The ends of marriage dimension also showed a strong relationship with the population ethics dimension. Pleasure was not treated by the respondents as a consistent dimension, but was related either to questions of safety or of morality depending upon the specific question. The orientational values were quite independent of the questions dealing with moral values, even those dealing with the naturalness of oral contraception.

One of the central findings of this study was an illustration of value factors at the scientific stage. A scale made up of items designed to measure judgments about the morality of contraception correlated significantly with a scale made of items designed to measure beliefs about the technical facts. This illustrates the contention that there is either bias and distortion (Type IIc) or selection of "important" information (Type IId) at the scientific stage.

Next we examined a group of items designed to measure clinical decisions made in medical practice (the application stage). We found that these decisions were closely related to both moral judgments and beliefs about the technical facts. They were less closely, but significantly related to certain items measuring the man/nature orientational value. We argued that our physicians were apparently avoiding the dangers of applying their scientific knowledge without regard to their moral beliefs (the engineering model), but were in danger of incorporating their own evaluative beliefs into decisions which affect the lay actor in those cases where there was not some systematic method of assuring that the lay actor's system of evaluation was compatible with the professional's.

Turning to the sociological background variables, we found that while parents' and respondent's religious affiliation were the most closely associated with the morality, technical, and application scales, they were far from perfect predictors. We argued that the use of religious affiliation rather than direct measures of the cultural value complex will mean the loss of much of the predictive power of the measure. Surprisingly, medical school sponsorship was not significantly related to religious affiliation of the respondent and was a poor predictor of the scales. Hospital affiliation was somewhat better than medical school affiliation, but still poor in comparison to religious affiliation of parents or respondent. Obstetrician-gynecologists were more likely to take positions favoring oral contraception as were younger physicians. No significant relationships were found relating the sex or geographical areas to the position of the physician.

Finally, we compared our results with those of Spivack in 1957 on two questions common to both studies. We found major changes in the direction of willingness to introduce the subject of contraception to pre-marital patients and child-spacing to postpartum patients who do not first bring up the subject.

This study illustrates many of the ways in which values are incorporated into one particular scientific and technological area of decision-making. It is hoped that the same theoretical concepts developed in Part I of this study will be of

use in the similar analysis of other areas of scientific and
technological decision-making.   In the next and final chapter,
we shall examine physician decision-making in a particular community in greater depth.   Here we shall attempt to compare the
views of the community's physicians to a group of their patients.

CHAPTER VII

[1]The preliminary form was also administered to 60 non-physicians and from the results the discriminatory power of each question was calculated according to the method of critical ratios described by Green and modified by Adorno. See Bert Green, "Attitude Measurement," in *Handbook of Social Psychology*, ed. by Gardner Linzey, (Cambridge, Mass.: Addison-Wesley Publishing Company, 1954), p. 351, and T. W. Adorno, *et al.*, *The Authoritarian Personality* (New York: Harper, 1950), pp. 76-83.

[2]Most items had six possible choices ranging from agree strongly to disagree strongly. Some of the multiple choice items had seven or eight choices. In these cases, the number was reduced to six by combining response categories in a manner which would eliminate some of the smallest groups.

[3]Mary Jean Cornish, Florence A. Ruderman, and Sydney S. Spivack, *Doctors and Family Planning* (New York: National Committee on Maternal Health, Inc., 1963), p. 72.

[4]*Ibid.*, pp. 72-76. Very briefly, Low Catholic City is a West Coast community which is a major port, a processing, trading, and shipping center. High Catholic City is an Eastern manufacturing city with a high proportion of foreign born. Low Catholic Towns is actually a county in an Eastern state with old towns and some farming areas. High Catholic Towns is a collection of several small towns with surrounding farmlands comprising two counties in another Eastern state. It is an educational center with five colleges in the area. The two rural areas are both made up of five contiguous counties. Low Catholic Rural is primarily farmland in a Mid-Western state with soybeans, corn, poultry, and dairy being most important. High Catholic Rural, in another Mid-Western state, has a higher proportion of foreign born. Farming is more oriented toward dairy and cheese-production.

[5]*1969 American Medical Directory*, twenty-fifth edition (3 vols.; Chicago: American Medical Association, 1969). This includes physicians indicating specialization whether or not they have passed the specialty board. The directory contains a record of whether or not specialty boards have been passed. We did not ask this on the questionnaire, having plans to use the published information. We realized, however, that we stated in our cover letter that identification numbers would be used only to check returns and thus felt obliged to cancel plans for the correlation of directory information with the returns. Through the records in the *Directory*, we were able to exclude from our sample all those who were retired, interns and residents, or full-time teachers or administrators.

[6]We excluded those who specified general practice as a secondary specialty and some other area as primary. Those whose primary area was general practice and second area was obstetrics-gynecology were included in the first group. In order to have a workable group, Spivack took a one-third sample of the general practitioners in the cities. We followed the same procedure, but took fifty percent of them instead. The proportion of general practitioners to specialists had changed so drastically in the intervening period that this modification was necessary. In both his case and our own, when we make comparisons between groups, we shall weight the returns from these groups to reflect their true numbers. It should be pointed out that it is impossible to have anything but an arbitrary ratio of specialists to general practitioners in a sample in the first place. Not only has the proportion changed, but the roles of the two groups have changed. At both time points almost certainly the specialists are more active and influential in distributing birth control information than their general practice counterparts. In any comparisons between the two groups, this must be taken into account.

[7]Twelve additional respondents were unavailable, their questionnaires returned marked "moved," "addressee unknown," or "deceased."

[8]Alan F. Guttmacher, "Conception Control and the Medical Profession," *Human Fertility*, XII (March, 1947), p. 2.

[9]Cornish, *Doctors and Family Planning*, p. 78. In addition to using a professional research organization and interviewers, Spivack also had the cooperation of the County Medical Societies and an advisory committee of well-known men in the field whose names appeared on his introductory letter. These professional techniques were beyond the budgetary resources of the present study.

[10]As mentioned above, a few items had more than six response categories. These were recorded to reduce their number to six. Two items in the technical scales permitted the respondent to make a numerical estimate (one of a pregnancy rate, another of a side-effect rate). These were divided into six approximately equal groups for recoding. Approximately half of the items were statements with implications critical of oral contraception; the other half statements in favor. This is a standard questionnaire technique to avoid systematic biases by "negative" or "positive" attitudes on the part of respondents. Those items which had negative implications as stated were inverted for the purposes of producing a consistent scale. The directionality of the item was determined by content analysis and confirmed in each case by the sign of the correlation coefficient as compared to the rest of the items in the scale.

[11]Taking the mean of a number of items when there is one or more blanks will produce a biased mean if the blank item has a mean for all responses to that item which differs from the mean of all responses to the other items in the scale. Although

this procedure of taking a mean ignoring blanks is often done, it can bias the score for those with blanks on some items. In order to test this factor during the pre-test data processing, we actually calculated a weighted predicted score for each blank in each scale. This was done by determining the mean of all responses to that item and the mean on the scale for the respondent leaving one item blank. Then comparing his scale score with the scale scores of the rest of the sample, we were able to calculate a predicted response for the item left blank. This was an extremely tedious procedure and in no single case did this change the scale score significantly. This procedure was abandoned for the final data analysis.

[12]*The Data-Text System: A Computer Language for Social Science Research* (Cambridge, Mass.: Harvard University, 1967).

[13]A better way to empirically establish scales is by the factor analysis of the items in the instrument. We performed a factor analysis and a varimax factor rotation making use of the Data-Text computer program for these operations (*The Data-Text System*, pp. 265-84). The complete table of rotated factor loadings is reproduced in Appendix IV. The results of this procedure are somewhat ambiguous. Five factors were generated. The items are grouped according to factor in Appendix V. All items with factor loadings greater than .300 for the factor are listed. It is apparent that the items from the six scales of our cultural value complex grouped into three factors (2, 3, and 4). Of these, factor 4 is closely related to the value-orientational items and will be discussed below. Factor 3 includes all of the items from the promiscuity, natural morality, ends of marriage, and general morality scales with the single exception of item 42 which had been placed in the ends of marriage scale. This item, "To be fair to the other children, a couple has a moral obligation to try to limit pregnancies by a means as reliable as the pill," has a loading on factor 3 of .201, but the family-size element in this item was so dominant that it loads primarily onto factor 2. In addition, one item from the safety scale (item 49) has a high factor loading onto factor 3. This item which deals with the risks of side effects is an illustration of the close interaction between technical and ethical judgments which we shall discuss below. Finally, two items from the pleasure scale (items 18 and 46) and seven of the items from the application scale (items 51, 54, parts 2, 4,5,6,7 and 55) also have loadings onto factor 3 which are higher than .300. We shall discuss these interactions in the appropriate sections below.

Factor 2 is the other factor which incorporated many of the morality scale items. The common element in items loading onto factor 2 was that of population and family size. It incorporated all of the items from the population morality scale plus three items from the ends of marriage scale which had a strong component of family size in them. Thus, the ends of marriage scale was an important element in factors 2 and 3. Factor 2 also incorporated two items dealing with population facts (items 17 and 43), one item from the pleasure scale (item 46), and two items from the application scale (items 54,

248

part 1, and 58). Here again, there is evidence of close interaction between the moral and other dimensions. This will be
discussed below.

Ideally, we would have performed a second level of factoring. This was our original intention. A factoring limited to
the evaluative items presumably would have differentiated the
ethical and other evaluative factors more clearly. Unfortunately, there was no computer time available for this second
level of factoring.

[14]Florence R. Kluckhohn and F. L. Strodtbeck, *Variations
in Value Orientations* (Evanston, Ill.: Row, Peterson, 1961).

[15]The calculations supporting this statement are quite
complicated. All of the value orientational items were scored,
like the other items, on a scale from plus three (agree strongly) to minus three (disagree strongly). Since the mean for the
items was not the same, the scores were not comparable in the
initial form. To generate comparable data, we calculated the
Z scores. Then for the nature dimensions we divided the respondents into three groups: man over nature group (those with
the man over nature item Z score higher than the score on the
nature over man item and also higher than the man in harmony
with nature item), nature over man group, and a man in harmony
with nature group. The statistical procedures assured that we
would end up with three approximately equal groups each of
which tended to emphasize one of the three possible orientations on the relation of man to nature. Since the dimension
of the relationship of man to nature is not a linear one (some
will prefer the position of man in harmony with nature over
either extreme), ordinal scaling techniques could not be used.
We thus generated three nominal scales which could be cross-
tabulated with the morality scales. In order to do this, the
morality scales were divided into four approximately equal
groups. The same procedure was carried out for the three-time
orientation items (13, 19, and 28).

CHAPTER VIII

THE PHYSICIAN AND HIS PATIENT: A COMMUNITY STUDY

In the last chapter we presented a study of physicians'
views drawing our sample from several parts of the country and
using techniques which, while easily codified, do not permit
the depth of understanding and subjective feelings which would
be helpful. In particular, we were not able to examine the
views of the lay actors (patients) in relationship to those of
their physicians. In our theoretical discussion in the first
part of this volume we developed the concepts of "the consensus
of expert opinion" and a series of models for the lay-professional relationship. We suggested that unless it could be assumed that professionals, as a group, had a cultural value complex which was similar to that of laymen, the consensus of the
expert opinion may reflect a systematically skewed value perspective. We also suggested that unless one can assume that
the individual professional's cultural value complex in the
area under consideration resembles that of the layman with whom
he is dealing, there are dangers in the "clinical model" of
lay-professional relationships. The professional may be incorporating a value system into his advice and decision-making
which is incompatible with the value system of the layman.

In this chapter we shall make a very preliminary attempt
to explore these questions. We have undertaken a study of one
community in a depth impossible in the larger scale, more quan-
titatively oriented survey of physicians reported in the last
chapter. In this community study we sought to accomplish three
things. Our objective was first to obtain a more subjective,
personal perspective through the intensive interviewing of a
group of physicians. This supplements interviews conducted in
the developmental phase of the research and is reflected
throughout our report. Second, we wanted to provide a preliminary comparison of the views of a coherent group of physicians
with a patient population which plausibly could be compared
with them. Third, we sought to make a preliminary examination
of the relationship of the views of specific patients with the
particular physicians they have selected.

While several writers have suggested the obvious importance of the physicians in patient decisions about contraception,[1] to our knowledge there is only one study which reports
actual examination of patients paired with their own physicians
and this consisted entirely of subjective reporting of the observation of an unspecified number of physicians "in the Pre-
natal Clinic of a large metropolitan hospital" together with an
unspecified number of "spot" interviews and examination of the
"records and follow-ups of over 300 clinical psychiatric interviews."[2]

A. THE METHOD OF THE COMMUNITY STUDY

For this portion of our research, we selected a group of
towns unrelated to the other phases of our work. The area has
as its center a town of approximately 39,000 people quite removed physically and psychologically from any larger metropolitan area. It includes seven contiguous townships in an Eastern
state. It was settled in the late seventeenth century and until recently was known for a large men's clothing industry.
More recently, diversified light industry including textiles,
electrical equipment, chemical, and metal products have been
the basis of its economy. The area was ideal for the type of
study we wanted to undertake because the group of seven townships made up the southern half of one of the state's official
"health service areas." The area has only one hospital, the
one around which the study was developed. There is a small
hospital serving the five townships making up the northern half
of the health service area, but there is little overlap between
the two areas. Only a minor amount of health care is obtained
from outside of the area. The entire area which draws medical
services from the central hospital had a population of approximately 72,000 in 1960. It is also interesting for the purposes of this study because it is somewhat more than fifty percent Catholic.

We carried out intensive interviews with all the obstetricians who use the town hospital and all the general practitioners who practice obstetrics. We were assisted in this phase of
our study by a physician in the area (who has no obstetrical

practice). We were both members of a group conducting a study
on population for the National Commission on Population Growth
and the American Future. We related the work reported here
into our preliminary research and fact finding for that study.
All physicians and patients were informed that we were clearly
involved in work which would eventually lead to a report to the
Population Commission. After preliminary meetings with the appropriate hospital authorities, we arranged to interview the
medical personnel. Prior to the interview, each was asked to
complete the same questionnaire used in the major study reported in the last chapter. We also sent a slightly modified form
of the questionnaire to all of the women delivering babies at
the hospital during a period of twenty-four consecutive days
early in 1971. An additional group of questionnaires has been
sent to patients in order to increase the sample size, but responses have not been complete enough to include in the present
report. We obtained the consent of the physicians prior to
sending the questionnaires to the patients.

This phase of our work provides an interesting check on
sampling. We were able to interview all of the physicians
practicing obstetrics in the area. We made no effort to reach
general practitioners other than those with actual obstetrics
practices. This differs from our sample in the larger study in
that in the larger study we included a sample of all general
practitioners. We actually determined the ones to whom questionnaires would have been sent based on the listing in the
American Medical Directory. Ten physicians would have been included as having primary or secondary practices in obstetrics-
gynecology (two of whom were primarily general practitioners).
We found that, of these ten, eight were actually in practice in
the specialty. One, born in 1886, was retired (though not so
indicated in the directory). This suggests that retirement
could account for the smaller percentage return from older physicians in our mailed survey. Another physician was practicing
surgery. There was also one young obstetrician who had come to
the area within the past year who was not listed in the directory. This confirms a fact of which we were already aware;
some of the younger physicians were necessarily missed by our

sampling procedure. There were two other general practitioners whose practices, so we were informed, included obstetrics. These eleven physicians, all of whom we interviewed, accounted for all but two of the ninety-eight births during the period of our study. Of those two, one woman was a Jehovah's Witness who received special medical attention.

All of the physicians indicated a willingness to be interviewed and complete the questionnaires. Two physicians, both general practitioners, who together accounted for only five of the births during the period we were studying, had not completed their questionnaires by the time of the interview. We interviewed them with the understanding that they would complete the questionnaires and return them to us. Both indicated a willingness to complete the questionnaires, but they said they had not had time. There was nothing in the interview which would indicate any other reason for the delay. Their responses have not been included in the present analysis since they were not available in time for data processing. The results of our experience in this community confirms our judgment that non-respondents to our mailed questionnaires failed to respond due to the pressures of their professional responsibilities rather than for any other reason.

B. THE PROFESSIONAL'S VIEWS

The physicians with obstetrical practices in the towns which we are discussing had stronger reservations about the morality of contraception than did those of the areas surveyed by mail. This would be expected from what we know about the makeup of the community. Seven out of the group of eleven identified themselves as being affiliated with the Catholic Church. We have argued that religious affiliation is a good, but far from perfect, indicator of moral views. We found that the Catholic physicians in the group had views which ranged from serious reservations to endorsement of contraception as morally obligatory. Since we make no claims that either this community or the sample for our entire study is random, we do not believe that the fact that the reservations are stronger on the whole in this community will seriously affect our

conclusions. Our primary interest is in the relationship of
the physicians with a particularly relevant type of practice in
this community to a group of patients in the same community.

In spite of the fact that the physician population had
serious reservations about contraception, it was apparent that
their views were in a rapid state of flux. This is an illustration of the value feedback loop which we have discussed.
Three incidents will illustrate the kind of change which is
taking place. Among the obstetrician-gynecologists in the area
there has existed two group practices. One of these included
two of the physicians who had the most doubts about the morality of contraception and a liberal Jewish physician who not
only prescribed contraceptives freely, but was the only physician willing to perform abortions. The two physicians with
reservations about prescribing oral contraceptives and insert-
ing IUD's would, in certain cases, refer their patients to
the Jewish physician. A combination of change in attitude on
the part of the two more hesitant physicians and pressure from
the more willing prescriber has brought about the dissolution
of the group practice, within the last year. Since that time
these two physicians have begun prescribing oral contraceptives. One has begun to insert IUD's although the potential
abortifacient action of the IUD had previously caused him to
refuse.

The second incident grew out of the first. One of these
two physicians, who has been in practice in the area longer
than any of the other obstetricians, seems to function as an
opinion leader. When he was faced with the need to prescribe
contraceptives himself he, in his words, "got hold of the
Bishop" and discussed with him the possibility of morally prescribing artificial means of contraception. He expressed that
he saw so many patients who seemed to need this and began to
doubt what harm it would do. He claimed, "I am a good Catholic; I stick by the rules." He said it was now his understanding that, while the Church can not condone artificial means as
a whole, each new case is unique and must be decided individu-
ally. He said he now thought that the pill was permissible to
use by "deserving couples" provided that they both agree and

that it was not their primary intention to avoid having any children. He now believes that morally he can write the prescription and the patient must decide whether to use it or not.

The third incident is the case of a young physician who was trained as a Catholic and had once written a thesis in a European Catholic school on the immorality of any artificial means of contraception. After an internship in a large metropolitan hospital where he was the only one not prescribing contraceptives, he is, according to his own account, "in a period of evolution as far as the moral standards are concerned." He said previously he would refuse to tell a patient where knowledge about contraception could be obtained. Now he holds the view that "people should form their own consciences." He said he now believes he should tell patients where they can get information they want. He claims that "the IUD is my gray zone now."

Of the themes of the morality factor of the cultural value complex, the physicians showed great concern for the use of the pill by the unmarried, especially by young girls. One who was obviously struggling to reach an ethical decision, responded when asked about prescribing for a sixteen year old girl, "That gives me alot of trouble....Don't give it to them right away. ...Try to reason with them....Get them to think it over."

They also showed great interest in the population theme, but their positions were complex. That they generally held that there was not an immediate problem can in part be accounted for by the small town atmosphere surrounding them. There is still much open space in the countryside. This was mentioned often in the interviews. Very frequently, however, the need to restrict growth in the lower income groups would come up. We incorporated several opportunities for physicians to freely express themselves during the course of the interview. This was done with very open-ended questions such as "Was there anything that came to mind from the questionnaire which you would like to comment on?" or "What do you think are some of the problems connected with birth control?" Often at these points the necessity for the lower class to restrict its procreation was introduced.

One physician who had a generally favorable attitude about contraception showed great willingness to encourage what he called "selective breeding." This could start, he said, with encouraging more use of contraception, but he said he thought eventually someone would have to say, "I'm sorry, you can't have any more children."

Before turning to the relationship of the views of the patients to those of the physicians, we should note in passing the patterns in the physicians' questionnaire responses. We find a general pattern consistent with the findings in the last chapter. There was a close relationship between the moral judgments of the physicians and the beliefs about the non-evaluative facts as measured by the technical scale. Both of these, in turn, were closely related to the application scale score. In Table 13 we list the rank order of each physician on each of these scales. It is apparent that the pattern is consistent.

TABLE 13

RANK ORDER OF PHYSICIAN SCALE SCORES

Physician Number	Morality Scale	Technical Scale	Application Scale
1	1	2	3
2	2	4	1
3	3	1	4
4	4	3	2
5	5	5	5
6	6	6.5	6
7	7	8	7
8	8	6.5	9
9	9	9	8

C. THE RELATIONS OF PATIENTS' AND PHYSICIANS' VIEWS

As mentioned above, we sent a slightly modified form of our questionnaire to the ninety-one patients who gave birth during the twenty-four consecutive days early in 1971[3] who were attended by one of the nine physicians for whom we had a completed questionnaire. In order to administer the questionnaire

to the patients some editing was required. The instructions
were changed so that they asked patients to express their views
and "take a guess" at any that required technical knowledge.[4]
The only other changes were to change technical terms such as
thrombophlebitis and carcinoma to less technical equivalents
such as blood clots and cancer,[5] and to add a few items on the
methods of contraception used by the patient and related items.

Follow-up to reach non-respondents was undertaken approximately two weeks after the questionnaires were mailed. We
first tried to reach every patient by telephone. Those who
could not be reached were sent a post card. From the telephon-
ing, we discovered two women in the sample who said they could
not answer because of a language barrier and two whose phones
had been disconnected. At the time the data were processed, we
had received thirty-two responses, a thirty-five percent return. We could find no evidence that the non-respondents differed significantly from those who replied. From our telephone
conversations we found no hostility to the research although
some expressed that they were too busy to respond to the six-
page questionnaire. The original group of ninety-one included
fifty-eight percent who were Catholic. Of those who returned
their questionnaires, fifty-six percent were Catholic.

1. *The Relationship of Religious Affiliation.*

Before going on to examine the actual responses of the patients and their relationship to the responses of the physicians, we shall examine a sociological measure, religious affiliation. In order to examine this relationship we made a
dichotomous classification into Catholic and non-Catholic for
both patients and physicians. Using the original sample of
ninety-one patients, we calculated that the percentage of patients that we would expect to have selected a physician whose
religious affiliation was the same as their own based upon
sheer chance. From the percentage of patients and physicians
in the Catholic and non-Catholic groups, we would have expected
fifty-four percent of the patients to have been paired with a
physician in the same group. In fact, fifty-six percent were
paired this way. This strongly suggests that patients were not

using religious affiliation as a criterion of selection of
their physicians or at least they were not attempting to obtain
a physician whose religious group matched their own. We have
every reason to believe that patients would have had evidence
of the physician's religious affiliation in most cases. They
are in a small community in which such information would probably be readily available. In all but two cases, the surnames
of the physicians would have given a clear indication of his
religious affiliation.

2. *The Relationship of the Scale Scores of the Physician
    Sample to Those of the Patient Sample.*

Using the scales from the questionnaire as discussed in
Chapter VII, we calculated the scale scores on the morality,
technical, and application scales for each patient and physician. The mean scale score in each case is presented in Table
14. A brief explanation of the interpretation of these numbers
is in order. It will be recalled that for each scale item the
respondent could indicate responses ranging from strong disagreement (-3) to strong agreement (+3). Since approximately
half the items were statements favoring contraception and half
opposing, those which were opposing were inverted (i.e., the
signs were changed) for purposes of scoring. The inverted
items are marked with a (-) in the Appendix II. The scale
scores were then calculated by taking the mean. Thus a mean of

TABLE 14

PATIENT AND PHYSICIAN MEAN SCALE SCORES

	Physician	Patient
Morality Scale	.74	.44
Technical Scale	.77	-.23
Application Scale	.56	.27

(positive) three would mean that the person agreed strongly
with all of the statements favoring birth control and disagreed strongly with all of the statements opposing birth control. The physicians in our community study had a mean score
of .74.[6] In contrast, the patients who responded had a mean
morality scale score of .44. Due to the small size of the sample, this difference was not quite significant at the .05
level. We hope to extend this portion of the study in the future to further test the significance of this difference.

The physicians and patients showed even greater differences in their beliefs about the non-evaluative facts as measured by the technical scale. The physicians had a mean score
of .77 while the patients score was -.23. This difference was
significant at the .001 level using the two-sample t-test for
the difference of means without requiring the assumption that
the two populations have the same standard deviations, as described by Blalock.[7]

The implications of these findings are provocative. If it
were demonstrated that a group of acknowledged experts in a
particular area (in this case contraception) holds beliefs
about the non-evaluative facts in their field of expertise
which differ from the layman, the normal interpretation would
be that those with acknowledged technical expertise are "nearer
the truth" and the layman should modify his position accordingly. However, the comparison of the three patient scale means
with the three physician scale means reveals an interesting
pattern. In each case, whether on the morality, the technical,
or the application scale, the patient has a position less favorable to contraception. Unfortunately these observations are
clouded by the lack of significance in the morality scale difference. If the morality scale difference could be demonstrated to be a systematic and significant one and if we could combine this information with the correlation of morality scale
scores of physicians with their technical scale scores which we
demonstrated in Chapter VII, then it would be plausible to suggest that the consensus of expert opinion would change in the
direction of the beliefs about the non-evaluative facts held by
the layman if the basic values and the cultural value complex

of the scientific professionals as a whole more nearly approximate those of the general public. This haunting suggestion warrants much more thorough and systematic investigation.

3. *The Relationship of the Individual Patient to Her Physician.*

Although the relationship of the patient population's views to those of the physician population is important, of even more importance is the relationship of the individual patient to her own physician. It makes no difference whether or not there are systematic differences in the two groups as a whole when it comes down to the specific decision-making process which takes place in the interaction between the professional and lay actors in a specific context. In order to examine this specific relationship, we examined the individual scale scores of each patient when paired with her own physician. Using a matched pairs t-test, we tested the hypothesis that the mean difference between the patient score and the physician score was zero.[8] First testing the relation of the patient's beliefs about the non-evaluative facts to those of her physician, we found they differed significantly (p < .001). This is in line with what we found in comparing the mean scores of the two samples. In every case, with the exception of one physician, every patient held beliefs about the non-evaluative facts which were less favorable toward contraception than did her physician. In the case of the one physician, who objected to the pill strongly on both moral and technical grounds, all of his patients held more favorable views.

Next we compared the morality scale scores of each patient with those of her physician. Here we also found statistically significant differences. In ten cases, the patient's moral judgments were more favorable toward contraception than those of her physician, in twenty-two cases they were less favorable.

The importance of this finding cannot be overemphasized. It appears, at least in this case, that there exists no consensus on either moral or technical judgments between the physician and his patient. Reflecting upon the models for technological decision-making and the professional-lay relationship discussed in Chapter IV, we suggest that there are grave dangers in the clinical model in which the professional incorporates his own system of evaluation into the decision-making process. If the professional does not share a value consensus with the layman (which appears to be the case here), decisions will be made dependent upon values alien to the layman's own value system.

If, on the other hand, the engineering model is operating in which the professional makes decisions incorporating the value system of the layman without any reference to his own, he may be led into actions which violate his own moral and other values. The collegial model, in which the professional takes it upon himself to treat the layman as a colleague, would resolve this dilemma if there were adequate basis for assuming that a collegial relationship exists. Unfortunately, in many professional-lay relationships in the present day with the existing social structures and relationships, this is not always the case. If it is the case, we are led to one or both of two alternatives. Either the contractual model, in which the rights and responsibilities, privileges and obligations, of both professional and lay actor are spelled out implicitly or explicitly, must be adopted or there must be some systematic method of pairing professional and layman so that the assumption of a consensus of evaluative systems, of cultural value complexes, is warranted. Since the development of either solution to perfection is utopian, it seems plausible to move simultaneously toward both. Whether this can be done without jeopardizing the norm of scientific objectivity in the narrow sense of eliminating bias and distortion (the Type IIc value factor) remains to be seen.

[1]E.g., Keith P. Russell and Gitta Meier, "Family Planning in the Hospital Setting," *California Medicine* CX (February, 1969), 114-19.

[2]Sanford R. Wolf and Elsie L. Ferguson, "The Physician's Influence on the Nonacceptance of Birth Control," *American Journal of Obstetrics and Gynecology*, CIV, No. 5 (July 1, 1969), pp. 752-57. Cornelis B. Bakker and Cameron R. Dightman, in "Physicians and Family Planning, A Persistent Ambivalence," *Obstetrics and Gynecology*, XXV, No. 2 (February, 1965), 279-85, report the study of 109 physicians and 100 patients, but the patient study was on a group of women participating in a project studying the psychologic factors involved in the use of oral contraceptives and was not linked with the study of the physicians.

[3]We actually sent questionnaires to all ninety-eight women giving birth during that period. As mentioned above, two were attended by physicians not in our sample. The other five were attended by the two physicians whose questionnaires were not included in the data processing.

[4]The first paragraph of the instructions read: "This questionnaire is designed to find out the views of patients like yourself on birth control and some related items. Most of the questions require no medical knowledge at all. For the few that do, please take a guess indicating whether you think you agree or disagree with the statement. For each statement there is a set of six possible responses." The remainder of the instructions was identical to that in the physician questionnaire, the text of which is in Appendix I except that the last paragraph about responding with regard to the best drug available was omitted.

[5]Due to a slight typographical error in the reproduction of the questionnaire for the patients, item 29 was deleted in the data processing for both patients and physicians in this phase of the study.

[6]This means that the average response on all of the morality scale items was somewhat below the "agree slightly" response for the statements favoring birth control and vise versa for those opposing it. It does not mean that the person "agrees slightly with the pro-birth control position." That would be the error of assigning absolute meaning to data which are valid only for purposes of comparison.

[7]Hubert M. Blalock, Jr., *Social Statistics* (New York: McGraw-Hill Book Company, 1960), pp. 175-76.

[8]*Ibid.*, pp. 179-81.

QUESTIONNAIRE SENT TO PHYSICIANS

(Original mimeographed on both sides of paper)

On the following pages you will find a series of statements expressing opinions of the kind you might hear from persons around you. For each statement there is a set of six possible responses:

+1 Agree slightly   -1 Disagree slightly
+2 Agree   -2 Disagree
+3 Agree strongly   -3 Disagree strongly

You are asked to read each statement and then write a plus one (+1) if you agree slightly; a plus two (+2) if you just agree and so forth.

If you have doubt about any of the items, please make the choice that comes nearest your opinion and then circle the response to indicate your reservation. Some of the items are intentionally vague. Any comments you wish to make will be gratefully received. Please mark item numbers beside each comment.

In some cases your opinion may differ with respect to different oral contraceptive preparations. Please respond to the items with respect to what you consider to be the steroid combination and dosage form of choice, i.e., answer considering only the "best" oral contraceptive available.

1. When there are no medical contraindications, a physician should provide oral contraceptives to any woman who requests them. _____

2. The increased use of birth control "pills" by unmarried girls indicates a decline in American morality. _____

3. Setting aside questions of morality, the "pill" is one of the most convenient methods of birth control available and avoids much unpleasantness of other methods. _____

4. A woman has the right to interfere with her body chemistry in order to limit her offspring. _____

5. One of the ends of marriage is the production of offspring. Those who seek to avoid offspring without medical reason may be acting selfishly. _____

6. Oral contraception is perfectly safe where there are no specific medical contraindications. _____

7. It is morally necessary to adopt the small family norm as an essential principle for stabilizing the size of population.

8. Skipping one pill near mid-cycle in the twenty-day cycle greatly increases the chance of conception.

9. The use of the "pill" by unmarried women may be of concern to some, but I cannot honestly say that it bothers me.

10. The physician's role is to become a part of our great technology in which man is subduing nature.

11. It is morally preferable to limit birth control to natural means such as abstinence and rhythm.

12. If I were a clergyman with my religious and moral convictions, I would have to advise my parishioners not to use oral contraceptives.

13. People do not have enough respect for time-honored traditions these days. We should work hard to keep up those good things from the past.

14. There is some evidence that oral contraceptives produce cancer.

15. Although it may also be a source of pleasure, we should never forget that the production of children is one of the great responsibilities of the marriage bond.

16. I consider myself very much of an individual. I would rather work by myself than with a team or for someone else.

17. Technology could supply sufficient food for the world population for the next hundred years even if population continued to grow at present rates.

18. Life will be dramatically more pleasant if hormonal steroids or some other very reliable means of contraception are used after the desired number of children has been reached.

19. The past has gone and the future is too uncertain. It is best to give more attention to what is happening now in the present.

20. The interests of one's family override any obligations to society in determining family size.

21. Death rates from thromboembolic disease are substantially higher for women on the pill than for those of the same age not on the pill.

22. The physician can best be understood as nature's helper. He assists nature in its healing process. _____

23. I would favor a hospital policy which made oral contraceptives available to all clinic patients without regard to marital status. _____

24. Oral contraception interferes with one of the ends of marriage. _____

25. When it comes right down to it, there is a basic tendency toward evil in most men. _____

26. The population growth in the United States is one of the lowest for the developed countries of the world. _____

27. I would have to classify oral contraceptive therapy as a morally questionable "artificial" means of limiting conception. _____

28. It is important to make every effort to look to the future and find new ways of doing things to replace the old. _____

29. When there are no medical contraindications, a physician should provide oral contraceptives to any married woman who requests them. _____

30. Having several closely-spaced children makes life extremely unpleasant for a mother. _____

31. The forces of nature are awe inspiring. The physician best serves his function if he has respect for the complexity of the human body and counts on nature to do its own healing. _____

32. There is something unjust about a couple with three children and substantial family income choosing to have another child. _____

33. When one considers all the different side effects, one must conclude that oral contraceptives offer significant risks to a woman's health. _____

34. What I care about most is accomplishing things; I like to see results and think they are worth working for. _____

35. The possibility that the pill might lead to increased promiscuity raises moral questions about its widespread availability. _____

36. Oral contraception helps couples become morally responsible parents by assuring only wanted children will be born. _____

37. Sometimes I have at least a slight feeling that the use of the "pill" is tampering with an area which is not man's province.

_____

38. There is something unpleasant about having to take a pill daily as a means of conception control.

_____

39. It is not morally justifiable for any outside agency to infringe on a couple's right to have children.

_____

40. Skipping two pills on two consecutive days near mid-cycle greatly increase the chance of conception.

_____

41. Physicians who are concerned about basic moral values in a society are not likely to prescribe oral contraceptives.

_____

42. To be fair to the other children a couple has a moral obligation to try to limit pregnancies by a means as reliable as the pill.

_____

43. At present rates of world population growth, many of our natural resources will be depleted within the next hundred years.

_____

44. It would be desirable from a moral point of view to have a reliable contraceptive means which was natural rather than artificial.

_____

45. Chances of death from taking the pill are greater than chances of death from the rhythm method (including deaths from pregnancies which might result in each case).

_____

46. Large families tend to get more enjoyment out of life than small ones.

_____

47. In a time of population crisis it may be morally acceptable to have some state regulation or influence regarding the number of children a couple may have.

_____

48. Access to hormonal steroids for contraception should be carefully controlled in order to minimize promiscuity.

_____

Please mark in the space provided the one answer which most closely agrees with your opinion.

49. If both you and your patient had no moral objection to oral contraception, how often would you refuse to prescribe such therapy to normal patients because of the risks of side effects?

_____ Always   _____ Occasionally   _____ Very Rarely

_____ Very Often   _____ Infrequently   _____ Never

_____ Often

50. If one thousand women had used oral contraceptives
    for one year (or until they became pregnant), how
    many would you expect to have become pregnant by
    the end of the year?   _____

51. In a premarital examination, if the patient does
    not bring up the subject of contraception, how
    often do you?

    _____ Always   _____ Fairly Often

    _____ Very Often   _____ Occasionally

    _____ Often   _____ Never

52. Which of the following is closest to your guess of
    what happened to the population of the United
    States in 1969?   _____

    a. declined somewhat   e. increased 2%
    b. stayed about constant f. increased 5%
    c. increased 0.5%   g. increased 10%
    d. increased 1%   h. increased 20%

53. For normal patients, what would you estimate to
    be the percentage who quit using oral contraceptives
    during a period of one year because of side effects?

                                            _____ percent

54. Below are several typical responses to requests of
    patients for contraceptive information or materials.
    Below that, some typical patients are described. For
    each patient described indicate which would be your
    most likely response by placing the appropriate letter
    in the place provided. For each case assume there
    exists no specific contraindications.

    Responses: a. fulfill the request of the patient
               b. explain availability of other methods and
                  then fulfill the request of the patient if
                  she still desires it
               c. encourage use of other methods and then
                  fulfill her request if she still desires it
               d. refer her to another physician
               e. refer her to a clergyman
               f. refuse to fulfill her request

    Indicate your most likely response for the cases below:

    (1) A non-Catholic patient who requests instruction
        in the rhythm method.   _____

    (2) A sixteen-year old, unmarried girl requesting
        oral contraceptives.   _____

(3) A Catholic patient who requests instruction in the rhythm method. _____

(4) A Catholic patient who requests a prescription for oral contraceptives. _____

(5) A non-Catholic low-income woman with six children who requests instruction in the rhythm method. _____

(6) A non-Catholic patient who requests a prescription for oral contraceptives. _____

(7) A twenty-six year old, unmarried girl requesting oral contraceptives. _____

55. If your postpartum patients don't ask for advice on child-spacing, how often do you introduce the subject?

_____ Always   _____ Sometimes
_____ Almost always   _____ Hardly ever
_____ Very often   _____ Never
_____ Often

56. Compared with the rhythm method, how much more effective would you estimate oral contraceptives to be in preventing pregnancy?

_____ twice or less   _____ 100 times
_____ 10 times   _____ 250 times
_____ 25 times   _____ 500 times
_____ 50 times   _____ 1000 times or more

57. What is your guess of the extent to which a patient on oral contraceptives for a ten-year period would run the risk of serious or permanently damaging effects (such as carcinoma, sterility, thrombophlebitis, etc.).

_____ None   _____ Moderate
_____ Virtually none   _____ Serious
_____ Very little   _____ Extreme
_____ Little

58. If a woman with three children, good health, and substantial family income expresses a desire for further children, how likely would you be to suggest to her that population growth is a factor to be considered in family planning?

_____ Certain   _____ Unlikely
_____ Very likely   _____ Very unlikely
_____ Likely   _____ Certain not to

59. What was the sponsorship of the medical school you attended?

_____ Governmental   _____ Private Protestant
_____ Private nonsectarian _____ Private Jewish
_____ Private Catholic

60. What is the sponsorship of the hospital with which you are affiliated?

_____ Governmental   _____ Private Protestant
_____ Private nonsectarian _____ Private Jewish
_____ Private Catholic

61. What is your area of medical practice?

_____ General Practice   _____ Obstetrics-gynecology
_____ Internal Medicine   _____ Other (Specify:_____
                                              _____)

62. Religion: _____ Catholic
               _____ Jewish
               _____ Protestant (Denomination: _____)
               _____ Other (Specify: _____)

63. What is (was) the religion of your parents?

               _____ Catholic
               _____ Jewish
               _____ Protestant (Denomination: _____)
               _____ Other (Specify: _____)

64. What is your estimate of the strength of your religious affiliation?

_____ Very strong   _____ Moderate
_____ Strong   _____ Weak

65. Age: _____ under 35   _____ 55-64
         _____ 35-44   _____ 65 or over
         _____ 45-54

66. Sex: _____ Male
         _____ Female

Thank you very much for your help in this project.

APPENDIX II

QUESTIONNAIRE ARRANGED ACCORDING TO SCALES

Morality Scale

	Correlation: Item-to-Sub-Scale	Correlation: Item-to-Morality Scale	Correlation: Item-to-Technical Scale
General Morality Sub-Scale			
1. When there are no medical contra-indications, a physician should provide oral contraceptives to any woman who requests them.	.776**[1]	.646**	.337**
12. If I were a clergyman with my religious and moral convictions I would have to advise my parishioners not to use oral contraceptives. (-)[2]	.712**	.620**	.402**
29. When there are no medical contra-indications, a physician should provide oral contraceptives to any married woman who requests them.	.823**	.638**	.464**
41. Physicians who are concerned about basic values in a society are not likely to prescribe oral contraceptives. (-)	.625**	.404**	.315**

[1]** means p < .01.

[2](-) means that the sign of the response has been inverted for purposes of scoring.

Morality Scale Item with next highest item-to-sub-scale correlation:

	Correlation: Item-to-Sub-Scale	Correlation: Item-to-Morality Scale	Correlation: Item-to-Technical Scale
23. I would favor a hospital policy which made oral contraceptives available to all clinic patients without regard to marital status. (Promiscuity sub-scale)	.625**	.724**	.365**

Promiscuity Sub-Scale

2. The increased use of birth control "pills" by unmarried girls indicates a decline in American morality. (-)	.769**	.588**	.267**
9. The use of the "pill" by unmarried women may be of concern to some, but I cannot honestly say that it bothers me.	.721**	.560**	.328**
23. I would favor a hospital policy which made oral contraceptives available to all clinic patients without regard to marital status.	.821**	.724**	.365**
35. The possibility that the pill might lead to increased promiscuity raises moral questions about its wide-spread availability. (-)	.804**	.661**	.374**

	Correlation: Item-to-Sub-Scale	Correlation: Item-to-Morality Scale	Correlation: Item-to-Technical Scale
48. Access to hormonal steroids for contraception should be carefully controlled in order to minimize promiscuity. (-)	.794**	.611**	.390**

Morality Scale Item with next highest item-to-sub-scale correlations:

1. When there are no medical contra-indications, a physician should provide oral contraceptives to any woman who requests them. (General morality sub-scale)	.612**	.646**	.337**

Naturalness Sub-Scale

4. A woman has the right to interfere with her own body chemistry in order to limit her offspring.	.679**	.582**	.401**
11. It is morally preferable to limit birth control to natural means such as abstinence and rhythm. (-)	.740**	.588**	.327**
27. I would have to classify oral contraceptive therapy as a morally questionable "artificial" means of limiting conception. (-)	.770**	.661**	.358**
37. Sometimes I have at least a slight feeling that the use of the "pill" is tampering with an area which is not man's province. (-)	.732**	.671**	.612**

	Correlation: Item-to-Sub-Scale	Correlation: Item-to-Morality Scale	Correlation: Item-to-Technical Scale
44. It would be desirable from a moral point of view to have a reliable contraceptive means which was natural rather than artificial. (-)	.648**	.370**	.187**

Morality Scale Item with next highest item-to-sub-scale correlation:

12. If I were a clergyman with my religious and moral convictions, I would have to advise my parishioners not to use oral contraceptives. (-) General morality sub-scale)	.635**	.620**	.402**

Ends of Marriage Sub-Scale

5. One of the ends of marriage is the production of offspring. Those who seek to avoid offspring without medical reason may be acting selfishly. (-)	.674**	.565**	.307**
15. Although it may also be a source of pleasure, we should never forget that the production of children is one of the great responsibilities of the marriage bond. (-)	.629**	.455**	.348**
24. Oral contraception interferes with one of the ends of marriage. (-)	.746**	.615**	.342**

	Correlation: Item-to-Sub-Scale	Correlation: Item-to-Morality Scale	Correlation: Item-to-Technical Scale
36. Oral contraception helps couples become morally responsible parents by assuring that only wanted children will be born.	.633**	.549**	.346**
42. To be fair to the other children, a couple has a moral obligation to try to limit pregnancies by a means as reliable as the pill.	.641**	.559**	.412**

Morality Scale Item with next highest item-to-sub-scale correlation:

27. I would have to classify oral contraceptive therapy as a morally questionable "artificial" means of limiting conception. (-) (Naturalness sub-scale)	.555**	.661**	.358**

Population Morality Sub-Scale

7. It is morally necessary to adopt the small family norm as an essential principle for stabilizing the size of the population.	.739**	.495**	.369**
20. The interests of one's family override any obligations to society in determining family size. (-)	.637**	.357**	.255**

	Correlation: Item-to-Sub-Scale	Correlation: Item-to-Morality Scale	Correlation: Item-to-Technical Scale
32. There is something unjust about a couple with three children and substantial family income choosing to have another child.	.582**	.339**	.175**
39. It is not morally justifiable for any outside agency to infringe on a couple's right to have children. (-)	.696**	.464**	.295**
47. In a time of population crisis it may be morally acceptable to have some state regulation or influence regarding the number of children a couple may have.	.755**	.501**	.379**

Morality Scale Item with next highest item-to-sub-scale correlation:

27. I would have to classify oral contraceptive therapy as a morally questionable "artificial" means of limiting conception. (Naturalness sub-scale) (-)	.337**	.495**	.358**

Pleasure Scale	Correlation: Item-to-Pleasure Scale	Correlation: Item-to-Morality Scale	Correlation: Item-to-Technical Scale
3. Setting aside questions of morality, the "pill" is one of the most convenient methods of birth control available and avoids much unpleasantness of other methods.	.531**	.329**	.365**
-8. Life will be dramatically more pleasant if hormonal steroids or some other very reliable means of contraception are used after the desired number of children has been reached.	.652**	.466**	.384**
30. Having several closely-spaced children makes life extremely unpleasant for a mother.	.586**	.182**	.191**
=8. There is something unpleasant about having to take a pill daily as a means of conception control. (-)	.548**	.303**	.299**
46. Large families tend to get more enjoyment out of life than small ones.	.622**	.539**	.367**

Morality Scale Item with highest item-to-pleasure-scale correlation:

	Correlation: Item-to-Pleasure Scale	Correlation: Item-to-Morality Scale	Correlation: Item-to-Technical Scale
42. To be fair to the other children, a couple has a moral obligation to try to limit pregnancies by a means as reliable as the pill. (Ends of Marriage sub-scale)	.498**	.559**	.412**

Technical Scale

	Correlation: Item-to-Sub-Scale	Correlation: Item-to-Morality Scale	Correlation: Item-to-Technical Scale
Safety Sub-scale			
6. Oral contraception is perfectly safe where there are no specific medical contraindications.	.689**	.320**	.551**
14. There is some evidence that oral contraceptives produce cancer. (-)	.589**	.231**	.451**
21. Death rates from thromboembolic disease are substantially higher for women on the pill than for those of the same age not on the pill. (-)	.701**	.232**	.557**
33. When one considers all the different side effects, one must conclude that oral contraceptives offer significant risks to a woman's health. (-)	.729**	.409**	.636**

	Correlation: Item-to-Sub-Scale	Correlation: Item-to-Morality Scale	Correlation: Item-to-Technical Scale
45. Chances of death from taking the pill are greater than chances of death from the rhythm method (including deaths from pregnancies which might result in each case). (-)	.553**	.389**	.503**
49. If both you and your patient had no moral objection to oral contraception, how often would you refuse to prescribe such therapy to normal patients because of the risks of side effects?	.488**	.380**	.449**
53. For normal patients, what would you estimate to be the percentage who quit using oral contraceptives during a period of one year because of side effects?	.364**	.169*[1]	.318**
57. What is your guess of the extent to which a patient on oral contraceptives for a ten-year period would run the risk of serious or permanently damaging effects (such as carcinoma, sterility, thrombophlebitis, etc.)?	.645**	.399**	.594**

[1]* means p < .05.

Morality Scale Item with highest item-to-safety-sub-scale correlation:

	Correlation: Item-to-Sub-Scale	Correlation: Item-to-Morality Scale	Correlation: Item-to-Technical Scale
37. Sometimes I have at least a slight feeling that the use of the "pill" is tampering with an area which is not man's province. (-)	.546**	.671**	.612**

Effectiveness Sub-Scale

	Correlation: Item-to-Sub-Scale	Correlation: Item-to-Morality Scale	Correlation: Item-to-Technical Scale
8. Skipping one pill near mid-cycle in the twenty-day cycle greatly increases the chance of conception. (-)	.669**	.071	.350**
40. Skipping two pills on two consecutive days near mid-cycle greatly increases the chance of conception. (-)	.607**	.005	.245**
50. If a thousand women had used oral contraceptives for one year (or until they became pregnant), how many would you expect to have become pregnant by the end of the year?	.579**	.273**	.443**
56. Compared with the rhythm method, how much more effective would you estimate oral contraceptives to be in preventing pregnancy?	.472**	.150*	.253**

Morality Scale Item with highest item-to-effectiveness-sub-scale correlation:

Item		Correlation: Item-to-Sub-Scale	Correlation: Item-to-Morality Scale	Correlation: Item-to-Technical Scale
37.	Sometimes I have at least a slight feeling that the use of the "pill" is tampering with an area which is not man's province. (-) (Naturalness sub-scale)	.277**	.671**	.612**

Demographic Sub-Scale

Item		Correlation: Item-to-Sub-Scale	Correlation: Item-to-Morality Scale	Correlation: Item-to-Technical Scale
17.	Technology could supply sufficient food for the world population for the next hundred years even if population continued to grow at present rates. (-)	.688**	.460**	.499**
26.	The population growth in the United States is one of the lowest for the developed countries of the world. (-)	.578**	.238**	.400**
43.	At present rates of world population growth, many of our natural resources will be depleted within the next hundred years.	.677**	.514**	.450**
52a.	Which of the following is closest to your guess of what happened to the population of the United States in 1969?	.541**	.080	.303**
52b.	Which is closest to your guess of what happened to the population of the world in 1969?	.510**	.001	.242**

Morality Scale Item with highest item-to-demographic-sub-scale correlation:

	Correlation: Item-to-Sub-Scale	Correlation: Item-to-Morality Scale	Correlation: Item-to-Technical Scale
47. In a time of population crisis it may be morally acceptable to have some state regulation or influence regarding the number of children a couple may have. (Population sub-scale)	.409**	.501**	.379**

Application Scale

	Correlation: Item-to-Application Scale	Correlation: Item-to-Morality Scale	Correlation: Item-to-Technical Scale
51. In a premarital examination, if the patient does not bring up the subject of contraception, how often do you?	.760**	.449**	.316**

Indicate your most likely response for the cases below. (See Appendix I for the full question.)

	Correlation: Item-to-Application Scale	Correlation: Item-to-Morality Scale	Correlation: Item-to-Technical Scale
54. (1) A non-Catholic patient who requests instruction in the rhythm method.	.449**	.281**	.168**
(2) A sixteen-year old, unmarried girl requesting oral contraceptives.	.695**	.556**	.361**
(3) A Catholic patient who requests instruction in the rhythm method.	.389**	.207**	.070

	Correlation: Item-to-Application Scale	Correlation: Item-to-Morality Scale	Correlation: Item-to-Technical Scale
(4) A Catholic patient who requests a prescription for oral contraceptives.	.606**	.604**	.526**
(5) A non-Catholic, low-income woman with six children who requests instruction in the rhythm method.	.459**	.317**	.263**
(6) A non-Catholic patient who requests a prescription for oral contraceptives.	.584**	.525**	.447**
(7) A twenty-six year old, unmarried girl requesting oral contraceptives.	.654**	.580**	.298**
55. If your postpartum patients don't ask for advice on childspacing, how often do you introduce the subject?	.773**	.488**	.398**
58. If a woman with three children, good health, and substantial family income expresses a desire for further children, how likely would you be to suggest to her that population growth is a factor to be considered in family planning?	.465**	.492**	.248**

Morality Scale Item with highest item-to-application-scale correlation:

	Correlation: Item-to- Application Scale	Correlation: Item-to- Morality Scale	Correlation: Item-to- Technical Scale
23. I would favor a hospital policy which made oral contraceptives available to all clinic patients without regard to marital status. (Promiscuity sub-scale)	.617**	.724**	.365**

APPENDIX III

COVER LETTER SENT TO PHYSICIANS

108 Holden Green
Cambridge, Massachusetts 02138

Dear Physician:

I am engaged in a research project concerning physicians' attitudes about birth control in connection with a doctoral dissertation at Harvard University. It is recognized that the physician is a very important source of birth control information, but very little is known about his attitudes on the subject.

Would you help in this project by filling out the short questionnaire enclosed? It should take only a few minutes. A stamped return envelope is enclosed. Of course all replies will be held in strictest confidence. The identification number will be used only to check completeness of returns.

Thank you for your cooperation. Your help will aid me and provide new knowledge on this important subject.

Sincerely yours,

Robert M. Veatch

ROTATED FACTOR LOADINGS

(Orthogonal Varimax, Rotation by Variable)

Item No.	1	2	3	4	5	Communality
1	.157	.130	-.638	-.327	.087	.563
2	-.035	.134	-.560	-.209	.233	.430
3	.516	.104	-.168	-.037	.103	.318
4	.352	.050	-.593	-.026	-.019	.480
5	.078	.293	-.433	.051	.088	.290
6	.583	.147	-.096	-.174	.013	.401
7	.174	.736	-.081	-.087	-.137	.605
8	.166	-.031	.054	.053	.407	.200
9	.077	.222	-.456	-.438	.156	.479
10	.157	.266	-.040	-.334	-.329	.317
11	.166	.140	-.626	.208	-.018	.483
12	.246	.171	-.646	.257	-.045	.575
13	-.158	-.061	.205	.047	.086	.080
14	.553	-.013	-.102	.126	.111	.345
15	.081	.343	-.312	.247	.238	.340
16	-.087	-.151	.100	-.490	-.004	.281
17	.107	.612	-.191	.056	.046	.428
18	.367	.255	-.343	-.247	-.196	.417
19	.032	-.014	-.092	-.490	-.007	.250
20	.005	.536	-.086	.281	.059	.378
21	.518	.161	-.006	.006	.149	.317
22	.051	.030	.187	-.348	-.124	.175
23	.071	.206	-.676	-.328	.248	.673
24	.197	.198	-.519	-.014	.190	.384
25	-.062	-.008	.049	.156	-.234	.085
26	.098	.096	-.198	.217	.169	.134
27	.204	.222	-.601	.183	.039	.488
28	.123	.237	-.048	-.205	-.147	.137
29	.429	.070	-.629	-.089	-.030	.593
30	.223	.299	.022	-.315	.057	.242
31	-.172	-.082	.103	-.365	-.029	.181

Item No.	1	2	3	4	5	Communality
32	-.152	.574	-.074	-.118	.045	.374
33	.606	.171	-.157	.044	.202	.464
34	.031	.008	-.057	-.425	-.051	.187
35	.099	.130	-.597	-.050	.303	.477
36	.299	.369	-.376	-.220	-.220	.464
37	.494	.159	-.512	.147	.138	.573
38	.514	.030	-.128	-.009	.098	.291
39	.150	.485	-.143	.029	-.118	.293
40	.074	-.029	.060	.124	.179	.058
41	.338	.043	-.350	.126	.033	.255
42	.347	.574	-.201	-.230	-.151	.566
43	.180	.631	-.215	-.045	-.067	.483
44	.018	.034	-.367	.324	.240	.299
45	.331	.376	-.172	.095	.054	.293
46	.118	.467	-.334	.118	.159	.383
47	.137	.652	-.102	.028	.054	.458
48	.015	.084	-.628	.023	.385	.550
49	.325	.019	-.370	.070	-.077	.254
50	.264	.131	-.125	-.116	.257	.182
51	.050	.174	-.421	.155	.557	.545
52a	.165	-.172	-.148	.105	-.067	.094
52b	.047	-.107	-.095	.027	-.177	.055
53	.154	.232	-.030	.113	-.119	.105
54(1)	-.240	.375	-.248	.195	.187	.333
54(2)	.064	.222	-.485	-.272	.378	.506
54(3)	-.312	.287	-.228	.185	.196	.305
54(4)	.488	.097	-.584	.062	-.007	.593
54(5)	.086	.156	-.377	.179	.006	.206
54(6)	.525	.030	-.492	-.028	.062	.524
54(7)	.109	.057	-.686	-.220	.102	.544
55	.125	.246	-.378	.119	.576	.566
56	.111	.179	-.067	-.120	.113	.076
57	.513	.213	-.203	.123	.128	.381
58	-.062	.623	-.215	-.038	.030	.440
64	.006	.180	-.286	-.315	-.008	.214

Item No.	1	2	3	4	5	Communality
65	.039	.073	.122	-.260	-.475	.315
66	-.231	.135	-.153	-.002	-.095	.104
Specialty	-.167	.155	.119	.056	-.655	.498

FACTORS IN THE ORAL CONTRACEPTION QUESTIONNAIRE

A tabulation of all items with loadings greater than .300 based upon varimax rotations classified according to original scales. (See Appendix I for individual questions; see Chapter VIII for discussion.)

Factor I: Safety

Safety Items	Loadings
33	.606
6	.583
14	.553
21	.518
57	.513
45	.331
49	.325

Other Safety Items

56	.154

Other Items with Loadings onto Factor I Greater Than .300

37 Natural Morality	.494
29 General Morality	.429
42 Ends of Marriage	.347
4 Natural Morality	.352
3 Pleasure	.516
38 Pleasure	.514
18 Pleasure	.367
54(3) Application	.312
54(4) Application	.488
54(6) Application	.525

Factor II: Population and Family Size

Population Morality Sub-scale Items	Loadings
7	.736
47	.652
32	.574
20	.536
39	.485

Ends of Marriage Morality Sub-scale Items

42	.574
36	.369
15	.343

Ends of Marriage Items Below .300   Loadings

        24   .197
         5   .078

Other Items with Loadings onto Factor II Greater Than .300

        43 Demographic Facts   .631
        17 Demographic Facts   .612
        46 Pleasure   .467
        58 Application (Population)   .623
     54(1) Application   .375

Factor III: The Ethics of Contraception

    General Morality Sub-scale Items

        12   .646
         1   .638
        29   .629
        41   .350

    Promiscuity Sub-scale Items

        23   .676
        48   .628
        35   .597
         2   .560
         9   .456

    Natural Morality Sub-scale Items

        11   .626
        27   .601
         4   .593
        37   .512
        44   .367

    Ends of Marriage Sub-scale Items

        24   .519
         5   .433
        36   .376
        15   .312

Items from the Above Scales with Loadings Below .300

        42 (Ends of Marriage)   .201

Other Items with Loadings onto Factor III Greater Than .300

        18 Pleasure   .343
        46 Pleasure   .334
        49 Safety   .370
        51 Application   .421
     54(2) Application   .485

```
54(4) Application                              .584
54(5) Application                              .377
54(6) Application                              .492
54(7) Application                              .686
  55 Application                               .378
```

Factor IV: Value Orientations

Value Orientation Items

```
   16                                          .490
   19                                          .490
   34                                          .425
   31                                          .365
   22                                          .348
   10                                          .334
```

Value Orientation Items with Loadings Below .300

```
   28                                          .205
   25                                          .156
   13                                          .047
```

Other Items with Loadings onto Factor IV Greater Than .300

```
    1 General Morality                         .327
    9 Promiscuity                              .438
   23 Promiscuity                              .328
   30 Pleasure                                -.315
   44 Natural Morality                         .324
```

Factor V: Area of Specialization

```
   61 Area of Medical Specialization          -.655
   55 Application                              .576
   51 Application                              .557
   65 Age                                     -.475
    8 Effectiveness                            .407
   48 Promiscuity                              .385
54(2) Application                              .378
   10 Value Orientation                       -.329
```

Items with Loadings onto No Factors Greater Than .300

```
   13  Value Orientation
   25  Value Orientation
   26  Demographic Facts
   28  Value Orientation
   40  Effectiveness
   50  Effectiveness
   52a Demographic Facts
   52b Demographic Facts
   53  Application
   56  Effectiveness
   66  Sex
```

APPENDIX VI

STATEMENTS ON BIRTH CONTROL AND RELATED SUBJECTS

1930 Central Conference of American Rabbis, Annual Convention

The Catholic Church, Pius XI, Encyclical, Casti Connubii

The Lambeth Conference (Anglican), Resolutions 13 and 15

1931 The Federal Council of Churches, Statement by the Committee on Marriage and Home

Congregational Christian Churches, General Council

1946 Protestant Episcopal Church, General Convention

1947 Association of Reform Rabbis of New York and Vicinity, Resolution

Evangelical and Reformed Church, General Synod

1951 The Catholic Church, Pius XII, Address to the Catholic Society of Midwives

The Catholic Church, Pius XII, Address

Jehovah's Witnesses, official journal statement

1954 Augustana Evangelical Lutheran Church, "Responsible Parenthood"

1956 Greek Archdiocese of North and South America, Statement of Archbishop Michael

The Methodist Church, General Conference, "The Christian Family"

United Lutheran Church in America, Convention, "Summary Statements on Marriage and Family Life"

1958 The Catholic Church, Pius XII, Address to the Association of Large Families of Rome and Italy

Rabbinical Alliance of America (Orthodox), Statement

The Lambeth Conference (Anglican), "The Family in Contemporary Society"

Evangelical United Brethren Church, General Conference

1959 World Council of Churches, Ecumenical Study Group (Mansfield Report), "Responsible Parenthood and the Population Problem"

Union of American Hebrew Congregations, General Assembly

American Baptist Convention, Convention

United Presbyterian Church in the U.S.A., General Assembly

Protestant Episcopal Church, National Council

1960 Central Conference of American Rabbis, "Planned Parenthood and Overpopulation"

The Methodist Church, Board of Social and Economic Relations

The Methodist Church, General Conference

Presbyterian Church in the U.S., General Assembly

Evangelical and Reformed Church, General Council

United Church of Christ, Council for Christian Social Action, "Responsible Parenthood and the Population Problem"

1961 The Catholic Church, Pope John XXIII, Encyclical *Mater et Magistra*

National Council of the Churches of Christ in the U.S.A., General Board, "Responsible Parenthood"

Committee on Jewish Law and Standards (Conservative), "Statement on Birth Control"

Southern Baptist Convention, Christian Life Commission

Protestant Episcopal Church, General Convention, "Christian Marriage and Population Control"

1962 Evangelical United Brethren Church, General Conference

Society of Friends, Philadelphia Yearly Meeting

The United Presbyterian Church of the U.S.A., General Assembly

International Convention of Christian Churches (Disciples of Christ), Assembly, "Christian Responsibility and Population Problems"

Unitarian Universalist Association, General Assembly, Resolution 10, "Population"

Reformed Church in America, General Synod, "Divorce, Remarriage and Planned Parenthood"

1963 American Baptist Convention

Assemblies of God, Statement of the General Superintendent

The United Presbyterian Church of the U.S.A., General Assembly

1964 The Catholic Church, Allocution of Pope Paul VI to the College of Cardinals

Protestant Episcopal Church, General Convention

Lutheran Church of America, Convention, "Statement on Marriage and Family"

1965 The Catholic Church, "The Dignity of Marriage and the Family" in The Constitution of the Church in the Modern World

The Catholic Church, Allocution of Pope Paul VI to the Papal Commission on Problems of the Family, Population, and Natality

Union of American Hebrew Congregations, General Assembly

American Jewish Congress, Governing Council

1966 The Catholic Church, Majority Papal Commission Report

The Catholic Church, Allocution of Pope Paul VI to Members of the Italian Society of Obstetricians and Gynecologists

The Catholic Church, Minority Papal Commission Report

Unitarian Universalist Association, General Assembly, "World Hunger and Population Control"

Episcopal Church, House of Bishops, "Population, Poverty, and Peace"

American Lutheran Church, Commission on Research and Social Action, "Responsible Reproduction"

1967 Orthodox Patriarch Athenagoras, statement

Friends Committee on National Legislation

American Friends Service Committee, Department devoted to Population Planning

United Church of Christ, Council for Christian Social Action, "Population Control"

1968 The National Council of the Churches of Christ in the U.S.A., General Board, Statement

The Catholic Church, Pope Paul VI, Encyclical, *Humanae Vitae*

Disciples of Christ, Convention Assembly, Resolution No. 56

General Conference Mennonite Church

The United Methodist Church, General Conference, "Responsible Family Planning"

1969 The National Council of the Churches of Christ in the U.S.A., General Board, "Resolution on the Time of Famine"

The United Methodist Church, Council of Bishops

The United Methodist Church, Board of Christian Social Concerns, "Population Crisis"

The United Methodist Church, Board of Christian Social Concerns, "Responsible Parenthood"

The United Church of Christ, General Synod, "Hunger, Population, and World Development"

1970 American Friends Service Committee, Working Party of the Family Planning Committee, "Who Shall Live? Man's Control over Birth and Death"

? A.M.E. Zion Church, Bishops Quadrennial Message, "Birth Control, Parenthood, and Population"

? Lutheran Church in America, Executive Council, "Statement Concerning Family Responsibility and Population Control for Consideration by the Board of Social Ministry"[1]

---

[1]Many of these statements have never been published. They have been obtained from general assembly records, pamphlets, brochures, and typed manuscripts as well as more traditional published sources. In a few instances we did not have access to complete pronouncements. Three unpublished collections have been used as a nucleus for our research. These are "A Compendium of Statements collected by Dr. Richard M. Fagley, Executive Secretary, Commission of the Churches on International Affairs at the request of the World Council of Churches and the International Missionary Council indicating the various positions adopted by a number of Churches, Councils and other Christian groups in relation to Parenthood and the Population Problem," (mimeographed) 1960; "Church World Service Planned Parenthood Program, Statements of Churches Concerning Problems of Population Growth," compiled by the Department of World Development, Board of Christian Social Concerns, United Methodist Church, June, 1969 (mimeographed); and the invaluable files of the McCormick library of Planned Parenthood-World Population in New York.

WORKS CITED

BOOKS

American Medical Association. *American Medical Directory, 1969.* 25th ed. 3 vols. Chicago: American Medical Association, 1969.

Aristotle. *The Nichomachean Ethics.* I,7. Edited by Martin Oswald. Indianapolis: Bobbs-Merrill, 1962.

Bales, Robert F. *Interaction Process Analysis.* Cambridge: Addison-Wesley Press, 1950.

Bates, Ralph S. *Scientific Societies in the United States.* 3rd ed. Cambridge, Mass.: M.I.T. Press, 1965.

Baumgarten, Eduard. *Max Weber, Werk und Person.* Tübingen: Mohr, 1964.

Becker, Howard S.; Greer, Blanche; Hughes, Everett; and Strauss, Anselm L. *Boys in White: Student Culture in Medical School.* Chicago: University of Chicago Press, 1961.

Berger, Peter. *The Sacred Canopy.* Garden City, N.Y.: Doubleday, 1967.

_____, and Luckmann, Thomas. *The Social Construction of Reality: A Treatise in the Sociology of Knowledge.* Garden City, N.Y.: Doubleday, 1966.

Blalock, Hubert M. *Social Statistics.* New York: McGraw-Hill Book Company, 1960.

Bloom, Samuel. *The Doctor and His Patient.* New York: Russell Sage Foundation, 1963.

Boese, Franz. *Geschichte des Vereins für Sozialpolitik: 1872-1939.* Berlin: Duncker und Humblot, 1939.

Boguslaw, Robert. *The New Utopians.* Englewood Cliffs, N.J.: Prentice-Hall, Inc., 1968.

Brandt, Richard B. *Ethical Theory: The Problems of Normative and Critical Ethics.* Englewood Cliffs, N.J.: Prentice-Hall, Inc., 1959.

Burling, Temple; Lentz, Edith; and Wilson, Robert N. *The Give and Take in Hospitals.* New York: Putnam, 1956.

Calvin: Institutes of the Christian Religion. Edited by John McNeill. 2 vols. Philadelphia: The Westminster Press, 1960.

Comte, Auguste. *Cours de philosophie positive*. 4th ed. 6 vols. Paris: Bailliere, 1877.

_____. *The Positive Philosophy of Auguste Comte*. Translated by Harriet Martineau. 3 vols. London: Bell, 1896.

Cornish, Mary Jean; Ruderman, Florence A.; and Spivack, Sydney S. *Doctors and Family Planning*. New York: National Committee on Maternal Health, Inc., 1963.

Craemer, Willy de, and Fox, Renée C. *The Emerging Physician*. Stanford, Calif.: The Hoover Institution, 1968.

The Data-Text System: A Computer Language for Social Science Research. Cambridge, Mass.: Harvard University, 1967.

Davidson, Donald; Suppes, Patrick; and Siegel, Sidney. *Decision-Making: An Experimental Approach*. Stanford: Stanford University Press, 1957.

Durkheim, Emile. *The Elementary Forms of Religious Life*. New York: The Free Press, 1965.

Fox, Renée C. *Experiment Perilous*. Glencoe, Ill.: The Free Press, 1959.

Freeman, Kathleen. *Pre-Socratic Philosophers*. Cambridge: Harvard University Press, 1946.

Friedrichs, Robert W. *A Sociology of Sociology*. New York: The Free Press, 1970.

Friedson, Eliot. *Patients' Views of Medical Practice*. New York: Russell Sage Foundation, 1961.

From Max Weber: Essays in Sociology. Edited by Hans Gerth and C. Wright Mills. New York: Oxford University Press, 1958.

Garceau, Oliver. *The Political Life of the American Medical Association*. Cambridge: Harvard University Press, 1941.

Gilson, Etienne. *History of Christian Philosophy in the Middle Ages*. New York: Random House, 1955.

Harris, Richard. *A Sacred Trust*. New York: New American Library, 1967.

Hippocrates. Translated by W. H. S. Jones and E. T. Withington. Vols. I-IV. London: Heineman, 1923-1931.

Horowitz, Irving Louis, ed. *The Rise and Fall of Project Camelot*. Cambridge, Mass.: M.I.T. Press, 1967.

Hutcheson, Francis. *Introduction to Moral Philosophy in Three Books Containing the Elements of Ethics and Law of Nature*. Glasgow: Robert and Andrew Foulis, 1753.

Jordan, Edwin P., ed. *The Physician and Group Practice*.
Chicago: Year Book Publishers, Inc., 1958.

Kant, Immanuel. *Groundwork of the Metaphysic of Morals*. New
York: Harper and Row, 1964.

Kaufman, Arnold. *The Science of Decision-Making*. London:
Weidenfeld, 1968.

Kelman, Herbert C. *A Time to Speak: On Human Values and Social
Research*. San Francisco: Jossey-Bass, Inc., 1968.

Kluckhohn, Florence R., and Strodtbeck, F. L. *Variations in
Value Orientations*. Evanston, Ill.: Row, Peterson, 1961.

Köhler, Wolfgang. *The Place of Value in the World of Facts*.
New York: New American Library, 1966.

Koos, Earl. *The Health of Regionville: What the People Thought
and Did About It*. New York: Columbia University Press,
1954.

The Lambeth Conference: 1958. London: S.P.C.K. and Seabury
Press, 1958.

Locke Selections. Edited by Sterling P. Lamprecht. New York:
Charles Scribners Sons, 1928.

Luckmann, Thomas. *The Invisible Religion: The Problem of Religion in Modern Society*. New York: The Macmillan Company,
1967.

Lyden, Freat J.; Geiger, J. Jack; and Peterson, Osler. *The
Training of Good Physicians*. Cambridge: Harvard University Press, 1968.

Malinowski, Bronislaw. *Magic, Science, and Religion and Other
Essays*. Garden City, N.Y.: Doubleday and Company, Inc.,
1948.

Mandelbaum, Maurice. *Phenomenology of Moral Experience*.
Baltimore: The Johns Hopkins Press, 1955.

Marcuse, Herbert. *One-Dimensional Man*. Boston: Beacon Press,
1964.

Mayer, Frederick. *A History of Ancient and Medieval Philosophy*. New York: American Book Company, 1950.

Mechanic, David. *Medical Sociology: A Selective View*. New
York: The Free Press, 1968.

Merton, Robert King; Reader, George; and Kendall, Patricia L.,
eds. *The Student-Physician: Introductory Studies in the
Sociology of Medical Education*. Cambridge: Harvard University Press, 1957.

Moore, G. E. *Principia Ethica*. Cambridge, England: Cambridge University Press, 1966.

Mumford, Emily, and Skipper, J. K. *Sociology in Hospital Care*. New York: Harper and Row, 1967.

Noonan, John T., Jr., ed. *The Church and Contraception: The Issues at Stake*. New York: Paulist Press, 1967.

Office of Science and Technology. *Privacy and Behavioral Research*. Washington, D.C.: Executive Office of the President, 1967.

Ornstein, Martha. *The Role of Scientific Societies in the Seventeenth Century*. Chicago: University of Chicago Press, 1938.

Parsons, Talcott. *The Social System*. New York: The Free Press of Glencoe, Inc., 1951.

_____. *Societies: Evolutionary and Comparative Perspectives*. Englewood Cliffs, N.J.: Prentice-Hall, 1966.

Pepper, Stephen C. *The Sources of Value*. Berkeley: University of California Press, 1958.

Perry, Ralph Barton. *Realms of Value: A Critique of Human Civilization*. Westport, Conn.: Greenwood Press, Inc., 1954.

Plato. *The Republic*. New York: Charles Scribners Sons, 1928.

Poynter, F. N. L., and Keele, K. D. *A Short History of Medicine*. London: Mills and Boon, 1961.

Rainwater, Lee. *And the Poor Get Children*. Chicago: Quadrangle Books, 1960.

Ramsey, Paul. *Deeds and Rules in Christian Ethics*. New York: Charles Scribners Sons, 1967.

Rescher, Nicholas. *Introduction to Value Theory*. Englewood Cliffs, N.J.: Prentice-Hall, Inc., 1969.

Rosenthal, Robert. *Experimenter Effects in Behavioral Research*. New York: Appleton Crofts, 1966.

_____, and Jacobson, Lenore. *Pygmalian in the Classroom*. New York: Holt, Rinehart, and Winston, 1968.

Ross, W. D. *The Right and the Good*. Oxford: Oxford University Press, 1930.

Sigerist, Henry E. *A History of Medicine*. New York: Oxford University Press, 1961.

Sjoberg, Gideon, ed. *Ethics, Politics, and Social Research.*
Cambridge, Mass.: Schenkman Publishing Company, Inc.,
1967.

Stanton, Alfred H., and Schwartz, Morris S. *The Mental Hospital.* New York: Basic Books, 1954.

Sumner, William Graham. *Folkways: A Study of the Sociological
Importance of Usages, Customs, Mores, and Morals.* New
York: Dover, 1959.

Szasz, Thomas. *The Myth of Mental Illness.* New York: Harper,
1961.

Tillich, Paul. *Systematic Theology.* 3 vols. Chicago: University of Chicago Press, 1951-1963.

Troeltsch, Ernst. *Protestantism and Progress: A Historical
Study of the Relation of Protestantism to the Modern
World.* Boston: Beacon Press, 1958.

Webb, Wilse B. *The Profession of Psychology.* New York: Holt,
Rinehart, and Winston, 1968.

Westermarck, Edward. *Ethical Relativity.* Westport, Conn.:
Greenwood Press, Inc., 1932.

Wilson, Robert N. *The Sociology of Health: An Introduction.*
New York: Random House, 1970.

Wolf, Abraham, ed. *A History of Science, Technology, and
Philosophy in the 16th and 17th Centuries.* New York:
Harper, 1959.

ARTICLES

Albert, Ethel M. "The Classification of Values: A Method of
Illustration." *American Anthropologist,* LVIII (1956),
221-48.

American Medical Association Committee on Human Reproduction.
"The Control of Fertility." *Journal of the American Medical Association,* CLXXXIV (October 25, 1965), 462-70.

American Public Health Association, Governing Council. "Policy
Statements: The Population Problem." *American Journal of
Public Health,* IL (December, 1959), 1703-4.

"The American Sociological Society." *Papers and Proceedings,
Annual Meeting.* I (1906), 1-2.

Bain, Read. "Science, Values, and Sociology." *American Sociological Review.* IV (August, 1939), 560-65.

Bakker, Cornelius C., and Dightman, Cameron R. "Physicians and Family Planning: A Persistent Ambivalence." *Obstetrics and Gynecology*, XXV (February, 1965), 279-84.

Bates, James. "A Model for the Science of Decision." *Philosophy of Science*, XXI (1954), 326-39.

Becker, Howard. "Whose Side Are We On?" *Social Problems*, XIV (Winter, 1967), 239-47.

"Birth Control: Some Recent Orthodox Statements." *Eastern Churches Review*, II (1969), 69-70.

"Blacks Supported by Psychologists." New York *Times*, September 3, 1969, p. 34.

Blake, Judith. "Reproductive Motivation and Population Policy." *BioScience*, (March 1, 1971), pp. 215-20.

Bumpass, Larry, and Westoff, Charles F. "The Perfect Contraceptive Population." *Science*, (September 18, 1970), pp. 1177-72.

Burgess, Ernest W. "The Aims of the Society for the Study of Social Problems." *Social Problems*, I (1953), 2-3.

_____. "Values and Sociological Research." *Social Problems*, I (1953), 16-20.

Buxton, C. L. "The Doctor's Responsibility in Population Control." *Northwest Medicine*, LXV (February, 1966), 112-16.

Cain, Leonard D., Jr. "The AMA and the Gerontologists: Uses and Abuses of 'A Profile of the Aging: USA'." *Ethics, Politics, and Social Research*. Edited by Gideon Sjoberg. Cambridge: Schenkman Publishing Company, Inc., 1967, pp. 78-114.

"The Constitution of the Church in the Modern World." *The Church and Contraception: The Issues at Stake*. Edited by John T. Noonan. New York: Paulist Press, 1967, pp. 49-60.

Crowley, Ralph M., and Laidlow, Robert W. "Psychiatric Opinion Regarding Abortion: Preliminary Report on a Survey." *American Journal of Psychiatry*, CXXIV, No. 4 (October, 1967), 145-48.

Cunningham, A. J. "Physicians and Contraception." *Canadian Medical Association Journal*, XCII (January 9, 1965), 87.

Dahrendorf, Ralf. "Values and Social Science." *Essays in the Theory of Society*. Stanford: Stanford University Press, 1968, pp. 1-18.

"A Diabetes Tea Party Hits FDA." *Medical World News* (December 18, 1970), pp. 13-14.

Dodd, Stuart A. "On Classifying Human Values." *American Sociological Review*, XVI (1951), 645-65.

Duncker, Karl. "Ethical Relativity." *Mind*, XLVIII (1939), 39-56.

Edelstein, Ludwig. "Ethics of the Greek Physician." *Ancient Medicine: Selected Papers*. Baltimore: The Johns Hopkins Press, 1967, pp. 319-48.

_____. "The Genuine Works of Hippocrates." *Bulletin of the History of Medicine*, VII (1939), 236-48.

_____. "Greek Medicine--Religion and Magic." *Ancient Medicine: Selected Papers*. Baltimore: The Johns Hopkins Press, 1967, pp. 205-46.

_____. "The Hippocratic Oath: Text, Translation, and Interpretation." *Ancient Medicine: Selected Papers*. Baltimore: The Johns Hopkins Press, 1967, pp. 3-63.

Eliot, Johan W.; Hall, Robert E.; Wilson, J. Robert; and Houser, Carolyn. "The Obstetrician's View." *Abortion in a Changing World*. Robert E. Hall, editor. 2 vols. New York: Columbia University Press, 1970, I, 85-95.

Eliot, Johan W., and Meier, Gitta. "Fertility Control in Hospitals with Residencies." *Obstetrics and Gynecology*, XXVIII (October, 1966), 582-91.

Etzioni, Amitai. "On Public Affairs Statements of Professional Associations." *The American Sociologist*, III (November, 1968), 279-80.

Firth, Roderick. "Ethical Absolutism and the Ideal Observer." *Philosophy and Phenomenological Research*, XII, No. 3 (March, 1952), 317-45.

Fox, Herb. "SESPA: A History." *Science for the People*, II (December, 1970), 2-3.

Fox, Renée C. "Medical Scientists in a Chateau." *Science*, CXXXVI (1962), 476-83.

_____. "Some Social and Cultural Factors in American Society Conducive to Medical Research on Human Subjects." *Clinical Investigation in Medicine: Legal, Ethical, and Moral Aspects*. Boston: Boston University Law Medicine Research Institute, 1963.

_____. "Training for Uncertainty." *The Student-Physician*. Edited by Robert K. Merton, George Reader, and Patricia Kendall. Cambridge: Harvard University Press, 1957, pp. 207-43.

306

Friedson, Eliot. "The Organization of Medical Practice."
Handbook of Medical Sociology. Edited by Howard E. Free-
man, Sol Levine, and Leo G. Reeder. Englewood Cliffs,
N.J.: Prentice-Hall, Inc., 1963, pp. 299-320.

_____. "The Sociology of Medicine: A Trend Report and Bib-
liography." *Current Sociology*, X-XI, No. 3 (1961-62).

Frankena, W. K. "The Naturalistic Fallacy." *Readings in
Ethical Theory*. Edited by Wilfred Sellars and John Hospers. New York: Appleton-Century-Crofts, Inc., 1952.

Freedman, Ronald. "The Sociology of Human Fertility: A Trend
Report and Bibliography." *Current Sociology*, XI, No. 2
(1962).

Gilson, Etienne. "La Doctrine de la double verité." *Etudes de
philosophie medievale*. Strasbourg: Commission de Publication de la Faculté des Lettres, 1921, pp. 51-75.

Glazer, William A. "Medical Care: Social Aspects." *International Encyclopedia of the Social Sciences*, X (1968),
95-96.

Gordon, Theodore J. "The Feedback Between Technology and
Values." *Values and the Future*. Edited by Kurt Baier
and Nicholas Rescher. New York: The Free Press, 1969,
pp. 148-92.

Gouldner, Alvin W. "Anti-Minotaur: The Myth of Value-Free
Sociology." *Sociology on Trial*. Edited by Maurice Stein
and Arthur Vidich. Englewood Cliffs, N.J.: Prentice-Hall,
Inc., 1963, pp. 35-52.

_____. "The Sociologist as Partisan: Sociology and the
Welfare State." *American Sociologist*, III, No. 2 (1968),
103-16.

Green, Bert. "Attitude Measurement." *Handbook of Social Psychology*. Edited by Garner Linzey. Cambridge, Mass.:
Addison-Wesley Publishing Company, 1954.

Guttmacher, Alan F. "Conception Control and the Medical Profession." *Human Fertility*, XII (March, 1947), 1-10.

Hall, Oswald. "The Informal Organization of the Medical Profession." *Canadian Journal of Economics and Political
Science*, XII (1946), pp. 30-41.

_____. "Types of Medical Careers." *American Journal of
Sociology*, LV (1949), 243-53.

Hall, Robert E. "Therapeutic Abortion, Sterilization and Contraception." *American Journal of Obstetrics and Gynecology*, XCI (February 15, 1965), 518-32.

Hall, Robert E. "New York Abortion Law Survey." *American Journal of Obstetrics and Gynecology*, XCIII, No. 8 (December 15, 1965), 1182-83.

Halliday, R. J. "The Sociological Movement, the Sociological Society, and the Genesis of Academic Sociology in Britain." *Sociological Review*, XVII (1968), 377-98.

Henderson, L. J. "Physician and Patient as a Social System." *New England Journal of Medicine*, CCXII (1935), 819-23.

_____. "The Practice of Medicine as Applied Sociology." *Transactions of the Association of American Physicians*, LI (1936), 3-22.

Herndon, C. N. and Nash, E. M. "Premarriage and Marriage Counselling: A Study of Practices of North Carolina Physicians." *Journal of the American Medical Association*, XXCC (1962), 395-99.

"A History of the AAAS or You Been a Good Ole Wagon But You Done Broke Down." *Science for the People*, II (December, 1970), 15-16.

Hoffman, Lois. "How Do Good Doctors Get That Way?" *Parents, Physicians and Illness*. Edited by E. Gartley Jaco. Glencoe, Ill.: The Free Press, 1958, pp. 365-81.

_____. "The Insurgent Sociologist: Counter-Convention Call." *Insurgent Sociologist*. Berkeley, California, 1969.

_____. "John of Jandun." *Encyclopedia of Philosophy*, IV. New York: Macmillan Company, 1967, pp. 280-82.

John XXIII. "Mater et Magistra." Translated in "Minority Papal Commission Report," in *The Catholic Case for Contraception*. Edited by Daniel Callahan. New York: The Macmillan Company, 1969.

Johnson, J. Prescott. "The Fact Value Question in Early Modern Value Theory." *The Journal of Value Inquiry*, I (1967), 64-71.

Kagan, Richard. "McCarran's Legacy: The Association for Asian Studies." *Bulletin of Concerned Asian Scholars*, IV (May, 1969), 18-22.

Katz, Daniel. "Organization Effectiveness and Change; An Evaluation of SPSSI by Members and Former Members." *The Journal of Social Issues*, Supplement Series, No. 11, 1958.

Kim, Han Young. "Balance and Dissonance Theories of the Adoption and Diffusion of an Innovation Applied to the IUCD." *Social Biology*, XVII, No. 1 (March, 1970), 43-53.

Kluckhohn, Clyde and others. "Values and Value-Orientations in the Theory of Action." *Toward a General Theory of Action.* Edited by Talcott Parsons and Edward Shils. New York: Harper and Row, 1951, pp. 388-433.

Kruse, Cornelius. "Western Theories of Value." *Essays in East-West Philosophy.* Edited by C. A. Moore. Honolulu: University of Hawaii Press, 1951, pp. 383-97.

Lake, Alice. "The Pill." *McCalls* (November, 1967), pp. 96-97 *et passim.*

Landis, Judson. "Attitudes of Individual California Physicians and Policies of State Medical Societies on Vasectomy for Birth Control." *Journal of Marriage and the Family,* XXVIII (August, 1966), 277-83.

Leach, Edmund. "Lévi-Strauss in the Garden of Eden: An Examination of Some Recent Developments in the Analysis of Myth." *Reader in Comparative Religion: An Anthropological Approach.* Second Edition. Edited by William A. Lessa and Evon Vogt. New York: Harper and Row, 1965, pp. 574-81.

"Leftist Historians." Chicago *Tribune,* (January 2, 1970), p. 20.

Lévi-Strauss, Claude. "The Structural Study of Myth." *Structural Anthropology.* Garden City, N.Y.: Doubleday and Company, 1963, pp. 202-28.

Lief, Harold I. "Orientation of Future Physicians in Psychosexual Attitudes." *Manual of Contraceptive Practice.* Edited by Mary S. Calderone. Baltimore: Williams and Wilkins, 1964, pp. 104-19.

_____. "Sexual Attitudes and Behavior of Medical Students: Implications for Medical Practice." *Marriage Counseling in Medical Practice.* Edited by E. M. Nash, *et al.* Chapel Hill, N.C.: University of North Carolina Press, 1964, pp. 301-18.

Locke, John. "Essay Concerning Human Understanding." *Locke Selections.* Edited by Sterling P. Lamprecht. New York: Charles Scribner's Sons, 1928.

Luther, Martin. "An Open Letter Concerning the Hard Book Against the Peasants." *Works on Martin Luther,* IV. Philadelphia: Muhlenberg Press, 1931, pp. 259-81.

_____. *The Precious and Sacred Writings of Martin Luther.* Translated by John H. Lenker. ("Epistle Sermon, Twelfth Sunday After Trinity," Vol. IX; "Gospel Sermon, Twenty-Third Sunday After Trinity," XIV. XIV.) Minneapolis, Minnesota: Lutherans in All Lands, Inc., 1903-1910.

MacKinney, Loren C. "Medical Ethics and Etiquette in the Early Middle Ages." *Bulletin of the History of Medicine*, XXVI (January-February, 1952), 1-31.

"Majority Papal Commission Report." *The Catholic Case Against Contraception*. Edited by Daniel Callahan. New York: The Macmillan Company, 1969, pp. 49-173.

Merton, Robert K. "The Bearing of Empirical Research on Sociological Theory." *On Theoretical Sociology*. New York: The Free Press, 1967, pp. 156-71.

"Modern Medicine Poll on Abortion." *Modern Medicine* (November 3, 1969).

Nash, E. M. "Attitudes of Physicians Affecting Contraceptive Practice." *Manual of Contraceptive Practice*. Edited by Mary S. Calderone. Baltimore: Williams and Wilkins, 1964, pp. 96-103.

Nicolaus, Martin. "Remarks at the ASA Convention." *The American Sociologist*, IV (May, 1969), 154-56.

Parsons, Talcott. "An Approach to the Sociology of Knowledge." *Sociological Theory of Modern Society*. New York: The Free Press, 1967, pp. 139-65.

_____. "Definitions of Health and Illness in the Light of American Values and Social Structure." *Patients, Physicians, and Illness*. Edited by E. Gartley Jaco. New York: The Free Press, 1958, pp. 165-87.

_____. "Evaluation and Objectivity in Social Science." *Sociological Theory and Modern Society*. New York: The Free Press, 1967, pp. 86-87.

_____ and Fox, Renée C. "Illness, Therapy and the Modern Urban Family." *Patients, Physicians and Illness*. Edited by E. Gartley Jaco. New York: The Free Press, 1958, pp. 234-45.

_____. "Mental Illness and 'Spiritual Malaise.'" *Social Structure and Personality*. New York: The Free Press, 1964, pp. 292-324.

_____. "Pattern Variables Revisited." *Sociological Theory and Modern Society*. New York: The Free Press, 1967, pp. 192-219.

_____. "Research with Human Subjects and the 'Professional Complex.'" *Daedalus* (Spring, 1969), 325-60.

_____. "Some Theoretical Considerations Bearing on the Field of Medical Sociology." *Social Structure and Personality*. New York: The Free Press, 1964, pp. 325-58.

Paul VI. "Humanae Vitae, 'On Human Life.'" *The Catholic Case For Contraception*. Edited by Daniel Callahan. New York: The Macmillan Company, 1969, pp. 212-36.

Pepper, Stephen C. "A Brief History of General Theory of Value." *A History of Philosophical Systems*. Edited by Vergilius T. Ferm. New York: Littlefield, 1950, pp. 493-503.

Perkin, Gordon W. "Physicians and Contraception." *Canadian Medical Association Journal*, XCII (March 20, 1965), 631-32.

"Physicians and Contraception." *Canadian Medical Association Journal*, XCI (October, 1964), 820-21.

Pius XI. *Casti Connubii*. Translated in "Minority Papal Commission Report." The Catholic Case for Contraception. Edited by Daniel Callahan. New York: The Macmillan Company, 1969, pp. 174-211.

"Radicals Chide 'Uptight' Sociologists on the Coast." New York *Times*, (September 6, 1969), p. 25.

"Responsible Parenthood and the Population Problem: Report of a Special Ecumenical Study Group." *Eugenics Quarterly*, VI, No. 4 (December, 1959), 219-24.

Russell, Keith P., and Meier, Gitta. "Family Planning in the Hospital Setting." *California Medicine*, CX (February, 1969), 114-19.

Schatzman, Morton. "Madness and Morals." *Radical Therapist*, I (October-November, 1970), 11-15.

Scrimshaw, Susan C., and Pasquariella, Bernard. "Obstacles to Sterilization in One Community." *Family Planning Perspectives*, II, No. 2 (October, 1970), 40-42.

Sherwin, Lawrence, and Overstreet, Edmund W. "Therapeutic Abortion: Attitudes and Practices of California Physicians." *California Medicine*, CV (November, 1966), 337-39.

Siegal, Earl, and Dilleway, Ronald. "Some Approaches to Family Planning Counseling in Local Health Departments: A Survey of Public Health Nurses and Physicians." *American Journal of Public Health*, LVI (November, 1966), 1840-46.

Simey, T. S. "Max Weber: Man of Affairs or Theoretical Sociologist?" *Social Review*, XIV, No. 3 (November, 1966), 303-28.

Smith, Harvey L. "Two Lines of Authority." *Patients, Physicians and Illness*. Edited by E. Gartley Jaco. New York: The Free Press, 1958, pp. 468-77.

Smith, Nicholas M., Jr.; Walters, Stanley S.; Brooks, Franklin C.; and Blackwell, David H. "The Theory of Values and the Science of Decision: A Summary." *Journal of the Operations Research Society of America*, I (1953), 103-13.

"Social, Economic Basis for Abortion Upheld." *Medical Tribune*, (October 31-November 1, 1964), pp. 21-22.

Spengler, Joseph P. "Values and Fertility Analysis." *Demography*, III (1966), 109-30.

Spivack, Sydney S. "The Doctor's Role in Family Planning." *Journal of the American Medical Association*, CXCII (April, 1964), 152-56.

_____. "Family Planning in Medical Practice." *Research in Family Planning*. Edited by Clyde V. Kiser. Princeton: Princeton University Press, 1962, pp. 193-210.

Tietze, Christopher, *et al.* "Teaching of Fertility Regulation in Medical Schools. Survey of the United States and Canada, 1964." *Journal of the American Medical Association*, CXCVI, (April 4, 1966), 20-24.

"The Tolbutamide Debate." *Medical World News*, (January 8, 1970), 37-46.

Troeltsch, Ernst. "Das stoisch-christliche Naturrecht und die moderne profane Naturrecht." *Gesammelte Schriften*, IV. Tübingen: Verlag J.C.B. Mohr (Paul Siebeck), 1925, pp. 166-91.

Walton, John. "Discipline, Method and Community Power: A Note on the Sociology of Knowledge." "American Sociology of Knowledge." *American Sociological Review*, XXXI (1966), 684-89.

Ward, Lester F. "The Establishment of Sociology." *Papers and Proceedings*, *Annual Meeting*, I (1906), 3-9.

Weber, Max. "The Logic of the Cultural Sciences." *The Methodology of the Social Sciences*. New York: The Free Press, 1949, pp. 113-88.

_____. "The Meaning of 'Ethical Neutrality' in Sociology and Economics." *The Methodology of the Social Sciences*. New York: The Free Press, 1949, pp. 1-47.

_____. "Objectivity in Social Science and Social Policy." *The Methodology of the Social Sciences*. New York: The Free Press, 1949, pp. 49-112.

Weiskotten, Herman G., *et al.* "Trends in Medical Practice--an Analysis of the Distribution and Characteristics of Medical College Graduates, 1915-1950." *Journal of Medical Education*, XXXV (1960), 1071-1121.

Wessan, Albert F. "Hospital Ideology and Communication Between Ward Personnel." *Patients, Physicians and Illness.* Edited by E. Gartley Jaco. New York: The Free Press, 1958, pp. 448-68.

Wilson, Robert N. "Patient-Practitioner Relationship." *Handbook of Medical Sociology.* Edited by Howard E. Freeman, Sol Levine, and Leo G. Reeder. Englewood Cliffs, N.J.: Prentice-Hall, Inc., 1963, pp. 273-95.

_____. "Teamwork in the Operating Room." *Patients, Physicians and Illness.* Edited by E. Gartley Jaco. New York: The Free Press, 1958, pp. 491-501.

Willson, J. P. "The Physician's Responsibility in Family Planning and Population Control." *Michigan Medicine*, LXIV (May, 1965), 332-34.

Wolf, Sanford R., and Ferguson, Elsie L. "The Physician's Influence on the Non-acceptance of Birth Control." *American Journal of Obstetrics and Gynecology*, CIV, No. 5 (July 1, 1969), 752-57.

Wood, H. C. "Medical Responsibility in Solving Population Problems." *Pacific Medicine and Surgery*, LXXIV (July, August, 1966).

Young, Stephen Grant. "Parent and Child: Compulsory Medical Care Over Objections of Parents." *West Virginia Law Review*, LXV (1963), 184-87.

Zbrowski, Mark. "Cultural Components in Response to Pain." *Journal of Social Issues*, VII (1952), 16-30.

Zda, I. "Problems of Communication, Diagnosis, and Patient Care." *Journal of Medical Education*, XXXV (1963), 829-38.

UNPUBLISHED DOCUMENTS

Barnes, John; Johnson, Larry; Kaufman, Helen; Nichols, William; and Olsson, Peter. "Attitudes and Practices of Physicians Concerning Birth Control in Two California Counties." (unpublished manuscript, 1965)

"Birth Control, Parenthood and Population." Bishops Quadrennial Message, A.M.E. Zion Church, undated. Text is on file at the Planned Parenthood-World Population Library, New York.

Bokser, Rabbi Ben Zion. "Statement on Birth Control." Final Draft Approved by the Committee on Jewish Law and Standards. (Unpublished manuscript, January 31, 1961).

Burch, G. "The Use of the Proper Theoretical Models in the Scientific Study of Religion." (unpublished paper, 1970).

Central Conference of American Rabbis. "Planned Parenthood and Overpopulation." Text is on file at the Planned Parenthood-World Population Library, New York.

Dyck, Arthur J. "A Gestalt Analysis of the Moral Data and Certain of its Implications for Ethical Theory" (unpublished Ph.D. dissertation, Harvard University, 1965).

Easterlin, Richard. "The American Baby Boom in Historical Perspective." Bureau of Economic Research, 1962.

Eastern Union of Radical Sociologists. "Open Letter to Colleagues." July, 1969.

Egan, Gerard. "Contractual Approaches to the Control and Modification of Behavior in Encounter Groups" (unpublished paper presented at the 1970 meetings of the American Association for the Advancement of Science).

Eliot, John W.; Stack, John; Smith, Roy; and Sullivan, Patricia. "Michigan Physicians' Views on Changing Michigan Abortion Laws and Experience with Abortion Requests" (unpublished manuscript).

Evangelical United Brethren Church. "Resolution on Responsible Parenthood of the General Conference, 1962" (unpublished manuscript). Text is on file in the Planned Parenthood-World Population Library in New York.

Fagley, Richard M., Collector. "A Compendium of Statements." (mimeographed, 1960)

National Council of Churches of Christ in the U.S.A., General Board. "Responsible Parenthood." (pamphlet, February 23, 1961)

People's Science Collective, New University Conference. "Science for the People" (mimeographed and distributed at the American Association for the Advancement of Science meeting in Chicago in December, 1970).

Protestant Episcopal Church, General Convention. "Christian Marriage and Population Control, 1961." Text is on file in the Planned Parenthood-World Population Library in New York.

Rabbinical Alliance of America. "Statement, 1958." Text is on file at the Planned Parenthood-World Population Library in New York.

Reformed Church in America, General Synod. "Divorce, Remarriage, and Planned Parenthood" (pamphlet, June, 1962).

Spivack, Sydney S. "Religious Attitudes of Physicians and Dissemination of Contraceptive Advice" (unpublished Ph.D. dissertation, Columbia University, 1959).

314

United Methodist Church, Board of Christian Social Concerns. "Statement of Churches Concerning Problems of Population, June, 1969" (mimeographed).

_____. "Population Resolutions" (pamphlet including resolutions on "population crisis" and "responsible parenthood" adopted October 6-9, 1969).

"Watch Tower." Official Journal of the Jehovah's Witnesses, March 1, 1951. Text is on file at the Planned Parenthood-World Population Library in New York.

Yates, Wilson. "American Protestantism and Birth Control: An Examination of Shifts with a Major Religious Value Orientation" (unpublished Ph.D. dissertation, Harvard University, 1968).

HARVARD DISSERTATIONS IN RELIGION

published under the aegis of the

HARVARD THEOLOGICAL REVIEW

by

THE SCHOLARS PRESS

Harvard Dissertations in Religion publishes outstanding dissertations in the study of religion submitted to Harvard University for the Ph.D. or Th.D. degree. Nomination of dissertations for the series is normally by the departments or thesis committees to which they have been submitted. Volumes are reproduced directly from typescript provided by the authors.

Harvard Dissertations in Religion publishes outstanding dissertations in the study of religion submitted to Harvard University for the Ph.D. or Th.D. degree. The goal of the HDR is to make the work of promising scholars available expeditiously and inexpensively. The HDR is published under the aegis of the *Harvard Theological Review*.

Nomination of dissertations for the HDR is normally by the departments or thesis committees to which they have been submitted, although nominations from individual faculty members will also be considered.

Volumes in the HDR are reproduced directly from the typescript provided by the authors. Responsibility therefore rests with the individual author for the accuracy and consistency of style and typography.

Caroline Bynum
George Rupp